Monsters, Demons

and

Psychopaths

Psychiatry and Horror Film

Monsters, Demons
and
Psychopaths

Psychiatry and Horror Film

Fernando Espi Forcen

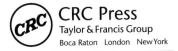

CRC Press
Taylor & Francis Group
Boca Raton   London   New York

CRC Press is an imprint of the
Taylor & Francis Group, an **informa** business

CRC Press
Taylor & Francis Group
6000 Broken Sound Parkway NW, Suite 300
Boca Raton, FL 33487-2742

© 2017 by Taylor & Francis Group, LLC
CRC Press is an imprint of Taylor & Francis Group, an Informa business

No claim to original U.S. Government works

Printed on acid-free paper
Version Date: 20160607

International Standard Book Number-13: 978-1-4987-1785-4 (Paperback)

Visit the Taylor & Francis Web site at
http://www.taylorandfrancis.com

and the CRC Press Web site at
http://www.crcpress.com

Printed and bound in the United States of America by
Edwards Brothers Malloy on sustainably sourced paper

This book is dedicated to my father who introduced us to his passion for the seventh art.

Contents

Preface

As long as I can remember, I've always loved horror. When I was a kid, my brothers and I had a special way of playing hide and seek. My father used to hide in one of the rooms of the house with the lights off and each one of us had to walk through the corridor not knowing where he was going to unexpectedly scare us. I remember with nostalgia the mixed feelings of fear, joy and excitement I experienced right before walking down the corridor. During my childhood, my cousins, my friends and I enjoyed telling each other horror stories about serial killers, urban legends or dangerous madmen that had escaped from the asylum. The first horror film I ever saw was *The Cabinet of Dr. Caligari*, a 1920 German silent movie. I was six years old and my father had told us that our grandfather was terrorized when he had watched it as a youngster. After watching the film I slept under the covers for at least a couple of weeks, scared by the feeling that the sleepwalker, Cesare, would come any minute to decide my fate.

One of those summers, while spending the holidays at a small town by the beach in Spain, my father shared with us the story of *Night of the Living Dead*, the 1968 movie which he had watched as a teenager and which was the scariest movie he had ever seen. Many years later during residency, together with my father, I visited the cemetery of Evans City, Pennsylvania, where several scenes had been shot.

Our caretaker at home, Moni, was in fact a horror film fan and she used to summarize for us the stories of *Alien*, *A Nightmare on Elm Street*, *Friday the 13th* and other classics. At that time our parents did not allow us to see those films and I had to wait for my teenage years. However, one night, when my twin brother Carlos and I were still children, my parents went out for dinner and left us in the care of my grandmother. That night, Stanley Kubrick's *The Shining* was playing on TV. My father had given instructions to my grandmother that she was not to allow us to see the film, something we were unaware of, but she fell asleep very quickly and we ended up watching that entire work of genius. I still remember my surprise when I watched the transformation from beauty to ugliness of the woman in Room 237.

I was eleven when I saw my first horror film in the theater: *Bram Stoker's Dracula* by Francis Ford Coppola. We sneaked into the theater, and the excitement and fear I felt was comparable to that I'd experienced as a kid right before walking down the dark corridor. I get a similar feeling every time I watch a new good scary movie now. I guess, at an early stage of development, I became somehow psychologically eroticized by horror and have been that way ever since. Today, at times when I am stressed, horror movies allow me to escape, relax and return to my happy upbringing.

I haven't just been fascinated by horror; cinema in general has been the one passion I inherited from my father. Despite going to a Catholic school in Murcia, in southeastern Spain, religion was not my thing. Luckily, in my school, the Marist Brothers were liberal enough. During my last year of high school, we were allowed to start a movie club as a substitute for catechism for those who were not interested in the sacrament of Confirmation. We worked under the supervision of Brother Soriano, who had studied cinema. Our movie club was poorly attended, though; most students were interested in receiving Confirmation. However, Brother Soriano helped us look at cinema in an academic way and opened our minds to new perspectives. I used the skills I had learned from Brother Soriano during medical school and designed a module for my classmates about cinema and medical psychology.

After medical school I left Spain to pursue a residency in psychiatry in the United States in Cleveland, Ohio. There I met Dr. Howard Gottesman who ran the movie club for the psychiatry residents. Every month the committee would select a film for psychiatric discussion among the residents. Dr. Gottesman taught us how to interpret films psychologically, a tool that has been fundamental to the development of this book. At that time I started to work with my twin brother on a paper about demonic possessions and mental illness in the Late Middle Ages. The paper was later published in the *Journal of Early Science and Medicine.* This would be the beginning of my Ph.D. on psychiatry and art history. Together we would later publish two more articles on demonic temptations in the Late Middle Ages in *The Journal of Nervous and Mental Disease* and *Palliative and Supportive Care.* Once I finished my residency I went to Chicago to do a fellowship in child and adolescent psychiatry. There, I started a new movie club and founded the *Journal of Humanistic Psychiatry*, which attempted to fill the gap in literature between psychiatry and humanities, including philosophy, history, art and cinema. The journal included a specific section for psychiatric discussion of films. By the end of my fellowship I proposed that my friends Susan Hatters Friedman and John P. Shand should submit to the 2014 American Psychiatric Association Annual Meeting in New York an innovative and unprecedented abstract. We agreed that "American Horror Film and Psychiatry" had great potential. Luckily our abstract was accepted and so were two papers on the theme that we wrote for *Australasian Psychiatry* and *The Lancet Psychiatry*. The presentation in New

York was well attended and later Lance Wobus, my editor at CRC Press, contacted me to write a book about psychiatry and horror film. Last year, I joined a new fellowship in psycho-oncology at Memorial Sloan Kettering while also writing this book. Sloan is a busy place to work and often I found myself setting the alarm for 5 a.m. to watch a horror film prior to going to work.

The knowledge and experience I have acquired during my personal journey through psychiatry, child and adolescent psychiatry, and psycho-oncology in the United States are directly and indirectly reflected in this book. The objective for this project has been to review the major horror films that have defined the genre, presented in a historical, sociological and cultural context. Methodologically, after an introduction to the film, a brief summary of the plot is presented to allow psychiatric interpretation of the different aspects of interest. The goal is to help the reader to discuss specific scenes, the development of characters and the narrative and connect them to psychiatric concepts. The reader will therefore be able to learn about the psychological interpretation of films as well as concepts of psychopathology and psychiatry. The approach to mental illness throughout history is also analyzed. The films are also viewed through historical, artistic and philosophical prisms. The book is written in an easy to read and at times humorous way, avoiding technical jargon, with the hope of reaching an audience relatively unschooled in our beloved field of psychiatry.

I would like to thank my family, friends, teachers, mentors and my editor for support, ideas and valuable feedback during writing. I hope you enjoy psychiatry and horror films as much as we do.

About the Author

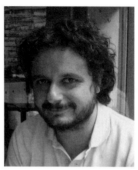

© Jill Krementz

Fernando Espi Forcen was born and raised in Spain. After graduating from medical school at the University of Murcia, he went to the United States to pursue a residency in psychiatry at MetroHealth Medical Center in Cleveland, Ohio. Subsequently he trained in child and adolescent psychiatry at the University of Chicago and completed a fellowship in psychosomatic medicine at Memorial Sloan Kettering Cancer Center in New York. Currently he is an assistant professor in the Department of Psychiatry of Rush University Medical Center in Chicago. He is the author of more than twenty peer-reviewed articles in different areas of psychiatry and the founding editor of the *Journal of Humanistic Psychiatry*, a quarterly online publication that combines psychiatry with humanities such as art, history and cinema. He also holds a Ph.D. with a thesis on the approach to mental illness in the Middle Ages.

Contact Information
Fernando Espi Forcen, M.D., Ph.D.
Assistant Professor, Department of Psychiatry, Rush University Medical Center
Professional Building, 1725 W. Harrison St., Suite 161
Chicago, IL 60612
Home address: 300 N State St Unit 3210, Chicago, IL 60654
Email: fespiforcen@gmail.com
Phone: +1 216 255 7219

CHAPTER 1

The Horror before Film

HUMANS HAVE ENJOYED HORROR since the beginning of civilization or perhaps even earlier. Before the "seventh art" of cinema was born, people enjoyed tales that provoke a somehow pleasurable panicky feeling of fear. According to Mesopotamian mythology, the gods created demons and monsters. For instance, Lamassus were human-headed winged oxen that guarded Assyrian palace doorways and gates to frighten away the forces of chaos. Lamashtu was a very fearful creature, represented with a lioness' head, a donkey's ears and teeth, and long fingers and fingernails, that preyed on unborn and newborn children. Pregnant women often wore an amulet depicting Pazuzu, who was charged with defending women and infants from Lamashtu. Pazuzu, a good demon, in addition to protecting pregnant women and their children, guarded humans against plagues and malevolent forces. Pazuzu was depicted with a monster's face and eagle claws. (Paradoxically, Pazuzu is the Mesopotamian demon that has taken possession of Regan in *The Exorcist*). According to the *Epic of Gilgamesh*, an epic poem from Mesopotamia and regarded as one of the earliest works of literature, the goddess Ishtar convinced her father to send the Bull of Heaven to kill people but Gilgamesh, king of Uruk, and his friend Enkidu were able to stop him. Earlier, the two friends had killed a giant with a hairy face called Humbaba who guarded Cedar Mountain.

Although we use the word "demons" to describe some of these counterparts of gods, etymologically the word "demon" comes from the Greek *daimon*, meaning a spirit. For the Greeks, however, these spirits could be good or bad. In Greek mythology, Typhon, the father of all monsters, was the most fearsome and deadly. He had a hundred dragon's heads erupting from his shoulders and neck. The female counterpart was Echidna, the mother of all monsters, represented as a half woman–half snake. Legendary hero Heracles had to kill the Nemean lion as one of his 'twelve labors' or penances. Cerberus was a multi-headed dog that guarded the underworld. While also an Egyptian monster, for the Greeks, the Sphinx had the body of a lion, the wings of a bird and the face of a woman and would kill anyone who could not solve her riddle. According to Sophocles' *Oedipus the King*, the Sphinx caused chaos in the city of Thebes until Oedipus solved the riddle. The Harpies were monsters with a female human face and the body of a bird that would steal food, and the Sirens were half woman–half bird monsters whose enchanting voice could cause ships to wreck on their island. Cyclops was a member of the race of giants and had only one eye. Medusa was a dreadful Gorgon with snakes as hair and a gaze that could turn anyone into stone. She was decapitated by Perseus with a mirror scythe. Another hero, Theseus, had to kill the Minotaur, a monster with the head of a bull and the body of a human, hiding in a labyrinth, in order to stop the human sacrifices ordered by King Minos.

In contrast to Greek beliefs about demons, Semitic civilizations referred to demons as merely bad spirits. As reported by the first book of Samuel in the Old Testament, future king David relieved the torments of Saul caused by a demon by playing the harp. As reported by the Gospels, Jesus believed in demonic possessions and practiced exorcisms. With the spread of Christianity in Europe, priests and other followers of Christ would also perform exorcisms as a way to imitate Jesus. During the Middle Ages, bestiaries were books that described the different actual or mythical animals and their behavior. These monsters were also often represented in the marginalia of books or in churches and cathedrals. One of these monsters was Donestre, a man with a lion's head who could speak every language. He was believed to approach random travelers and pretend that he knew their relatives in order to gain their confidence. Once the traveler thought he had found a good host Donestre would eat him and then mourn over his head. In medieval times, monsters were also depicted as regular humans with malformations or distorted anatomical features. For example, the head of Blemmyae was contained within their chest, and the Epiphagi had their eyes on their shoulders. The Troglodytes were very fast and did not talk. Gargoyles were elongated monsters that decorated the walls and served as waterspouts.

During the Late Middle Ages and especially in the Renaissance concern grew over witchcraft practice, especially the use of black magic. One alleged practice involved the turning of people into werewolves. The *Malleus Maleficarum* (Hammer of Witches), written in 1486, alerted the public to these kinds of practices and refuted arguments that witchcraft did not exist. Soon hysteria grew against these falsely accused witches all over Europe. Social outcasts, religious minorities and at times political rivals were accused of witchcraft practice, causing plagues and other calamities and unfortunately many were executed.

In the modern era, some Eastern Europeans have used theories of vampirism to explain the origin of plagues affecting small towns. With a lack of science and understanding of these problems, people craved for a magical explanation that could provide a quick solution. Rumors that dead people could come back to life with the intention of turning the living into vampires were common. Staking dead bodies with the hope of preventing more deaths in the community became a common practice. At this time too, when great ocean voyages led to the discovery of new lands and territories, sea monsters were used for decoration on maps.

It was mainly during the Romantic period of the nineteenth century that the so-called Gothic horror genre of literature rose to prominence. In 1818, Mary Shelley, while just twenty years old, published *Frankenstein: or, the Modern Prometheus* in England. Scottish author Robert Louis Stevenson published *The Strange Case of Dr. Jekyll and Mr. Hyde* in 1886, and Irish writer Bram Stoker published *Dracula* in 1897. On the Continent, in France in 1831 Victor Hugo published *The Hunchback of Notre-Dame*, while in Spain Gustavo Adolfo Bécquer was writing Romantic tales of the supernatural including "The Souls' Mountain" in 1861. In the United States, Edgar Allan Poe became the most prominent horror storywriter. His short story "The Black Cat" (1843) and narrative poem "The Raven" (1845) are among his most popular publications. Many of these Gothic horror novels were soon adapted into plays for theater and later were a major inspiration for the first silent films. In the period 1819 to 1823, acclaimed Spanish painter Francisco de Goya created some fourteen works known as his "Black Paintings" which depicted demonic possessions, witchcraft practice and body mutilation.

Finally, in 1896 pioneer French filmmaker George Méliès directed *Le Manoir Du Diable* (The Haunted Castle), considered to be the first horror film. In this silent film, a vampire bat turns into Mephistopheles (the Devil) and encounters several phantoms.

As we can see, people have long enjoyed tales of monsters, demons and horror, and horror has existed within art, literature and film throughout history.

CHAPTER 2

Silent Ḥorror

EXPRESSIONISM WAS AN ARTISTIC movement that started in Germany before World War I. As opposed to Impressionism – the prior leading artistic movement – which emphasized the importance of color and reflecting the immediate perception of the artist, Expressionism attempted to build more complex psychic structures, involving a distortion of the image in order to better express the inner quality of human emotion. The Expressionist movement was reflected in poetry, painting, architecture, dance and cinema. The birth of the German Expressionist movement took place in Dresden in 1905 with a group of artists who called themselves "Die Brücke" (The Bridge). Among them were Ernst Ludwig Kirchner, Fritz Bleyl, Karl Schmidt-Rottluff and Erick Heckel. The artists set up their studios in working class neighborhoods in an attempt to escape from the influence of the bourgeoisie and build "a bridge" to the art of the future. German Renaissance artists such as Matthias Grünewald, Lucas Cranach and Albert Dürer were their main influences. With the advent of World War I, Expressionism shifted towards a more rebellious protest against the devastation and negative impact that the war had made on society. Death, suicide, moral corruption, vice, and images of mutilated veterans became popular themes. Examples of this include Käthe Kollwitz's "Death Grabbing at a Group of Children," an image that revisits the medieval motif of the "Dance of Death"; Otto Dix's "The Match Seller," which portrays a homeless veteran, blind and limbless, sitting in the street selling matches, ignored by the well-heeled bourgeoisie while a dog is literally peeing on him; and George Grosz's "Suicide," in which the body of a suicide victim lies abandoned in the street in front of a brothel.

In cinema, German Expressionism focused on intellectual and macabre themes. The major directors of the time were Fritz Lang, Friedrich Wilhelm Murnau, Robert Wiene and Paul Wegener. The influence of psychiatry on their films is evident from their first motion pictures. Insanity became a recurrent topic such as in Robert Wiene's *The Cabinet of Dr. Caligari* (1920). The film had been initially offered to director Fritz Lang but he refused and Wiene was commissioned for the project in 1920. The idea of the movie had originated when writers Hans Janowitz and Carl Mayer met in Berlin after World War I. Both were enthusiastic about actor, writer and director Paul Wegener's early works (*The Student of Prague*, *The Golem*) and decided to write a horror film. They came up with the concept of telling the story of a psychiatrist and a somnambulist after visiting a nearby fair, where a man claimed to be able to predict the future during a hypnotic trance. As initially suggested by Fritz Lang prior to abandoning the project, the film's main character Francis narrates the film. Francis is a young man who attended the carnival of the German village of Holstenwall with his friend Alan. Both friends are competing for the love of the young and beautiful Jane. In the carnival they see the show of a psychiatrist and hypnotist named Dr. Caligari and a somnambulist, Cesare, in a coffin-like cabinet. As part of his show, Dr. Caligari induces a hypnotic trance in Cesare, which allows him to predict the future. An innocent Alan asks the somnambulist how long he shall live. Cesare's prediction is shocking: he will live only until dawn. That night, as the somnambulist had predicted, Alan dies at the hands of a shadowy figure. This crime will be just the first of a series of mysterious murders in the German village. Alan's friend Francis and Jane commence to investigate the murders and their research raises suspicions of Caligari and Cesare's relation to the homicides. When Dr. Caligari discovers the couple's intentions, he orders Cesare to kidnap and murder Jane. He creeps into Jane's home as she sleeps and is about to stab her but, overwhelmed by her beauty, abducts her instead. In the meantime, Francis goes to the local insane asylum to ask about Caligari and discovers through old records and a diary that Caligari, while still working as the head of the asylum, had become obsessed with an Italian monk who in 1703 had used a somnambulist to commit murder by proxy. This obsession led Caligari to attempt to prove whether it was in fact possible to do such a thing. After finding that Cesare is dead, Caligari reveals his insanity and is arrested by the authorities.

The original story written by Mayer and Janowitz intended to make clear that Caligari and Cesare were responsible for the crimes. However, the producers were interested in a less macabre ending and suggested that the film end with a twist in which a spectator unexpectedly discovers in the final scene that Francis is actually an inmate at the asylum and his story was the result of a delusion. In this alternative ending, the man who Francis called Caligari is actually the asylum director and he announces that, now that he understands Francis's delusion, he is confident he can cure his mental illness.

Three German Expressionist artists, Hermann Warm, Walter Reimann and Walter Röhrig, were hired to create the set design and props for the film. They produced a visual style with deliberate distortions of form, perspective and dimension. The oblique doors and chimneys, tilted roofs, arrow-like windows and trees, and the whole town of Holstenwall are reminiscent of the cities painted by the Expressionist Lyonel Feininger.

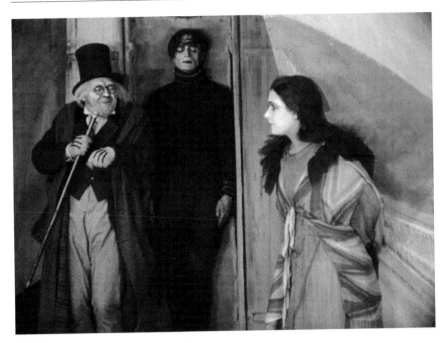

FIGURE 2.1 Dr. Caligari, The Hypnotist; Cesare, The Somnambulist; and Jane, The Object of Desire (*The Cabinet of Dr. Caligari*)

The legacy of *The Cabinet of Dr. Caligari* can still be seen in many contemporary movies. There are clear aesthetic parallels between Cesare and Edward in Tim Burton's *Edward Scissorhands* (1990). The twist ending or final revelation is now a common technique in cinema to maintain intrigue or surprise the spectator. David Fincher's *Fight Club* (1999) and Martin Scorsese's *Shutter Island* (2010) are great examples.

In the 1920s, psychopharmacology in psychiatry was not yet developed. Patients with severe mental illness were usually placed in insane asylums, in which moral treatment (a therapy that proposed a benevolent guidance for activities of daily living) was the standard approach. Hypnosis, a medical offshoot of Franz Mesmer's animal magnetism, was a valid therapy and patients with fantasies or delusions could be treated with hypnotherapy. In hypnosis, the hypnotist helps the subject fall into a sleep-like state with heightened suggestibility – a trance. As a result, the hypnotized person is able to focus on specific thoughts without being distracted by their surroundings.

In the late nineteenth century, while working at La Salpêtrière Hospital in Paris, renowned neurologist Jean-Martin Charcot supported the use of hypnosis for the treatment of hysteria (a syndrome that at the time was used to describe states of emotional excess with somatic symptoms, including neurological and psychiatric ones). Through hypnosis, a clinician could help patients enter a trance in which they would be more susceptible to queries about the true psychological nature of their symptoms. They could then potentially be cured through this self-awareness of the nature of their symptoms. Sigmund Freud learned hypnosis with Charcot in Paris and began practicing it. However, later he began thinking that hypnosis was too dependent on what the hypnotist suggested to the patient and proposed a free association technique in which a patient would lie on a coach and express random ideas that the clinician would carefully analyze during sessions. He called this method psychoanalysis. Nowadays hypnosis is still a valid therapy in psychiatry and has also been shown helpful in the treatment of anxiety, pain and insomnia and to help people increase concentration for studying. The works of Milton Erickson and Herbert Spiegel have been major influences on hypnosis in the United States.

There are several aspects of *The Cabinet of Dr. Caligari* that deserve our attention for a psychiatric discussion. In the first place, the film can be seen as a beautiful depiction of hypnosis and how it was portrayed at the time. Cesare is depicted as a highly hypnotizable person (usually just a very small percentage of the population have this quality). As a result he enters a highly suggestible trance state under Caligari's commands. The film uses psychiatric scientific literature to support what is happening. When Francis and three other physicians go to Caligari's office to investigate the crimes, they find a treatise on somnambulism published at the University of Uppsala in 1726. (In modern nomenclature, somnambulism is called sleepwalking disorder.) In this treatise, they learn about the case of the monk Caligari. In the asylum director's diary, they read about his obsession with the monk and his excitement at the prospect of a somnambulist possibly being admitted to the institution, giving him his opportunity to attempt to reproduce the monk's project. In a flashback, Dr. Caligari is depicted as going gradually insane surrounded by books on psychiatry right before leaving the asylum and he starts hearing voices saying, "You must become Caligari," which reveals the origin of the plot to the audience. After they bring Cesare's body to him, Caligari becomes enraged and attacks one of the physicians, requiring six people to restrain him, put him a straitjacket and secure him in a quiet room. At that time, chemical sedation was not possible and the straitjacket was the most common method of restraint. From a modern psychiatric point of view, Caligari could be seen as someone with bipolar disorder going into a psychotic mania, or an isolated psychotic episode. At this point the story would have ended, according to the initial script. However, in the alternative twist ending, we see Francis in the asylum yard with the rest of the patients, each one absorbed in their own delusion: an old man giving a speech on the stairs, a young woman playing an imaginary piano. Cesare is now seen stroking a bouquet and Jane believes she can't respond to Francis's advances because she has royal blood.

With the use of hypnosis at the beginning of the twentieth century, a debate took place in society over whether it was possible to make someone commit a crime under a hypnotic state. Charcot's disciple Gilles de la Tourette and forensic psychologist Hugo Munsterberg were inclined to believe that such a thing was not possible. Still, they acknowledged that it was something that could not be experimented with for obvious ethical reasons. The issue got more media attention when a female patient of Tourette's shot him in the head, alleging that she had been hypnotized without her consent. The debate over psychiatric treatment making someone commit a crime against their will still goes on today in similar ways. For instance, zolpidem is a sleep-inducing agent that has been associated with sleepwalking and has been used as an insanity defense in forensic settings. In recent times, Steven Soderbergh's film *Side Effects* (2013) narrates the story of a woman who unintentionally commits a crime after taking a drug prescribed by her psychiatrist.

After a failed attempt in 1915, with the help of architect Hans Poelzig and cinematographer Karl Freund, Paul Wegener filmed *The Golem: How He Came into the World* in 1920, a film that relates the story of the Jewish Rabbi Loew and the golem of Prague. The script was adapted from the 1915 novel *The Golem* by Gustav Meyrink. The film offers a masterly reproduction of the medieval Jewish ghetto with highly Expressionist scenery. The cinematography is considered one of the best achievements of German Expressionism. The film is set in the Middle Ages, and in the opening scene Rabbi Loew reads the stars and predicts a disaster for the Jewish community of Prague. The following day the Holy Roman Emperor sends one of his knights, Florian, to deliver a decree stating that Jews must abandon the city. The decree is a clear reference to the blood libel: "We can no longer neglect the complaints of the people against the Jews. They despise the holy ceremonies of Christ. They endanger the lives and property of their fellow men. They work black magic. We decree that all Jews shall be expelled from the city and all adjoining land before the end of the month."

Nonetheless, the arrogant knight has an immediate crush on the rabbi's daughter, Miriam, who seems to reciprocate his affections. In the meantime, with the assistance of Famulus, the rabbi creates a giant golem or anthropomorphic being out of clay. To bring him to life, they conjure the spirit of Astaroth, the crowned prince of Hell, who reveals the word "AEMAET." The rabbi writes the word and puts it in an amulet in the chest of the golem. This brings him to life. Initially, the golem is inoffensive and just performs domestic tasks for the rabbi in the ghetto. Later, Florian returns to the rabbi's house to bring an invitation to the upcoming Rose Festival. The rabbi brings the golem to the festival, producing excitement and terror in the audience of the court. After that the rabbi is asked to perform more magic. He then projects a magical screen showing the history of his people but first asks the audience not to laugh at it. After seeing an image of Ahasuerus, the wandering

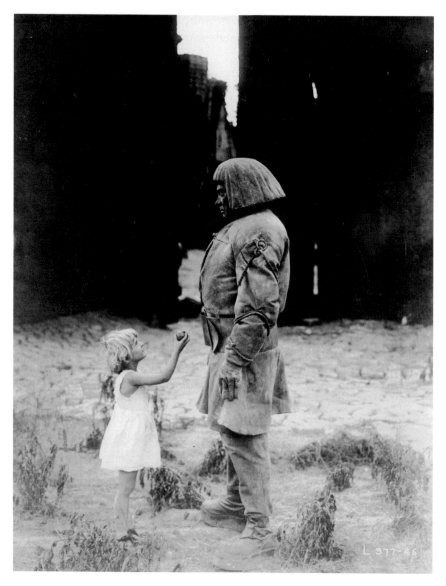

FIGURE 2.2 The Golem Facing the Innocence (*The Golem*)

Jew (who taunted Jesus during the passion and was made to walk for eternity), the audience, disregarding the rabbi's request, begins to laugh almost convulsively to the extent of making the palace collapse. However, the golem intervenes, saving the court. As a sign of gratitude for saving the palace, the emperor allows the Jews to stay in the city.

In the meantime, Florian and Miriam's romance continues, but Famulus, who is also interested in courting Miriam, finds out and becomes enraged, sending the golem to remove Florian from the ghetto. However, as the stars have continued to move, the golem is now under the evil influence of Astaroth, who instead throws Florian from the top of the tower, killing him. Then the golem sets the rabbi's house on fire and flees, taking Miriam with him by dragging her by the hair. When Rabbi Loew learns about the events he performs a spell to remove Astaroth from the golem, thus saving the community for a second time. A now docile golem leaves Miriam and breaks the gates of the ghetto and finds a group of children playing. All but a little girl run away. The golem holds the girl who innocently removes the amulet from his chest, making him collapse. When the rabbi and others find a lifeless golem, they pray and show gratitude for being saved for a third time within the same day.

According to traditional Jewish folklore, a golem is an anthropomorphic being created with the use of magic. The word "golem" appears only once in the Bible in Psalm 139:16: "Your eyes saw my golem; all the days ordained for me were written in your book before one of them came to be." Here, a golem refers to an unformed substance or an embryonic mass. The psalm has been interpreted as the connection between God and the creation of man, as God had conceptualized each one of us even before our own creation. The psalm has often been used to support the theory of determinism: we are at God's mercy and plans – no matter how much we try to plan our own life, life or God has plans for us.

The Jewish book *Sefer Yetzirah* or "Book of Creation" (third to fourth century AD) contains instructions on how to make a golem, with various rabbis commenting on different ways of making one. Most agree that the best way to make a golem is by creating a human-like figure and to bring it to life in the name of God (the ultimate creator).

In Ashkenazi Jewish lore, a golem may carry out tasks assigned by his creator and function as a servant. The most popular golem story is from Prague in the modern period. Rabbi Judah Loew ben Bezalel, the Jewish leader of Prague's ghetto (1513–1609) was said to have created a golem out of clay to protect the Jewish community from the blood libel against them. The blood libel or blood accusation became popular in Europe during the Middle Ages and modern period. It is a false accusation that Jews were committing terrible crimes against the Christian religion during their Jewish holidays, often killing children and using their blood in their religious ceremonies, contaminating wells to kill Christians, using profane images and desecration. Ever since the Gospels were written Jews were made guilty for the death of Christ. At first Christians did not dare to accuse the Romans of killing their Messiah for fear of being punished, so they accused the Jews instead: their rival creed in the expansion of Christianity throughout the empire. The role Jews played as tax collectors, physicians, king's counselors and other prestigious positions during the Late Middle Ages put them in a very delicate and dangerous situation. Their weak status as a religious minority allowed such accusations to be taken seriously, which unfortunately resulted in continual massacres of Jews throughout Europe over the centuries. During the Weimar Republic era, the film *The Golem* reflects the story of the blood libel and Jewish prosecution in Europe throughout the centuries. The golem also has interesting parallels with Mary Shelley's Frankenstein and even the more recent ghouls and zombies.

Among the film directors of the Weimar Republic era, Fritz Lang is perhaps the most celebrated. Lang was born in Vienna in 1890, studied civil engineering and art at the Technical University of Vienna, and combined his studies with his passion for art and painting. He traveled all over Europe before returning to Vienna to volunteer in World War I in which he was wounded three times. After his experience of being wounded in the war, he suffered from symptoms of what was then termed "shell shock" or "war neurosis," used to describe the neuropsychiatric manifestations that returning soldiers from combat experienced. After World War I and trench warfare, a "new" epidemic of this kind of post-combat stress was described. Initially, it was believed that shell shock was caused by combat-related concussive cerebral micro hemorrhages. However, symptoms were also described in patients with no exposure to physical trauma; therefore, the psychological stress of battle was proposed as a possible etiology of this condition. The term "shell shock" was widely accepted by the general population. However, in the medical and military literature the terms "neurasthenia" (usually given to higher ranks), "male hysteria" (usually given to lower ranks), and "nervous disease" were mostly used. The symptoms of shell shock implied inability to reason, walk or talk (as if the soldier was in a state of shock), symptoms that resemble another syndrome called catatonia (a final pathway of several mental disorders characterized by mutism, stupor and immobility with associated symptoms). Other symptoms of shell shock were fatigue, confusion, impaired hearing and vision, numbness, sleep problems, anxiety, mood swings, and impulsivity. This cluster of symptoms is today referred as posttraumatic stress disorder (PTSD), which usually happens after a life-threatening event such as combat, rape, accidents and so on. In fact, patients with PTSD can often go into a catatonic state.

As discussed earlier, World War I made a big impact on the subsequent expressions of art and cinema. Paranoia, fear of invasion, serial killers and mad scientists are central in Fritz Lang's films. He received international acclaim for his films about Dr. Mabuse, a psychoanalyst who uses his psychological knowledge to manipulate others for his own benefit. Mabuse is both an analyst and a hypnotist with telepathic powers to hypnotize people, as well as a master of disguise. Lang directed three films centered on this character through the decades. The first one, *Dr. Mabuse the Gambler* (1922), is based on the successful novel by Norbert Jacques, *Dr. Mabuse*. In the first scene, Dr. Mabuse has organized a theft to create panic and make profit on the stock market. Mabuse's mistress, Cara Carozza, under the analyst's instructions, seduces Edgar Hull, son of a millionaire industrialist, in order to have him play a card game in a gentlemen's club against a disguised Mabuse who subsequently hypnotizes him to play recklessly and lose heavily. As a result Mabuse makes a small fortune. In the meantime, state prosecutor Nobert von Wenk is investigating the felonies and goes undercover to a gambling den. Mabuse, in disguise, unsuccessfully tries to hypnotize the prosecutor and flees. At some point, Mabuse's mistress Carozza is imprisoned but she refuses to talk to protect the man she loves. Von Wenk places Countess Told in the same cell to see if she can help him get information by trickery; however, moved by Carozza's loyalty to her lover, the Countess refuses to assist von Wenk. In the interim, Dr. Mabuse, instead of making a plan to free his lover from jail, attends a séance where he meets Countess Told. Under hypnosis, she invites him to her house. There, he is entranced by her beauty, and to display his powers induces Count Told to cheat at poker. The other guests are outraged when they discover this, and the Countess faints. Mabuse uses this distraction to abduct her and carry her off to his lair. Thus ends the first part of the movie.

In the second part, Count Told visits Dr. Mabuse's office to seek help dealing with the fact that his wife is missing. This indeed is a perfect opportunity for Mabuse to ensure the Count does not learn of the Countess's whereabouts. Under Mabuse's treatment the Count goes insane and begins to suffer hallucinations. Meanwhile Mabuse orders his servant to poison Carozza while in jail to avoid possible betrayal. Mabuse also orders another of his henchmen, Pesch, to bomb von Wenk's office but he fails and is arrested. Fearing another betrayal, Mabuse arranges for Pesch to be shot and killed by a sniper while traveling on the police wagon. Finally, Mabuse then plans to leave the town and, infuriated by the Countess's refusal to go with him, uses his hypnotic powers to make the Count commit suicide in revenge. Von Wenk goes to Dr. Mabuse's office to interrogate him about the Count's mysterious suicide, as Mabuse is the Count's psychoanalyst. Mabuse suggests that he could have done it under the influence of a mass hypnotist called Sandor Weltemann and informs him that he should go and attend Weltemann's show. The mass hypnotist turns out to be Mabuse in disguise. During the show he hypnotizes von Wenk and makes him get in his car to drive off a cliff, but his men stop him at the very last moment. Realizing Mabuse's plans, von Wenk orders a siege of his house which results in a gunfight where Mabuse's men are either killed or arrested. After that, Mabuse flees underground to the workshop and becomes psychotic, seeing the ghosts of his victims. Finally the police find him at his workshop already insane and he is confined to an asylum. In the sequel, *The Testament of Dr. Mabuse* (1933), the analyst uses telepathic hypnosis from the asylum under a catatonic state to continue his misdeeds.

From a psychiatric point of view, Dr. Mabuse is portrayed as a man with antisocial personality disorder. His lack of empathy for others' suffering, his self-serving attitudes, cheating behaviors and difficulties with attaining the social norms would support the hypothesis. Dr. Mabuse is superficially charming in order to seduce and manipulate his victims, something characteristic of people with antisocial traits. On the other hand he ends up becoming psychotic and catatonic, a state that will continue in the second film of the saga. Individuals with antisocial personality often falsely claim to have psychotic symptoms (like hallucinations or delusions) in an attempt to offer an insanity defense, get drugs from physicians or excuse their actions. However, this does not seem the case for Dr. Mabuse. In the film he seems to fall into a legitimate psychotic state which leads him into catatonia. Like anyone else, people with antisocial personality disorder have at least a 1 percent risk of becoming psychotic or schizophrenic, which seems to be the case here. In *The Testament of Dr. Mabuse*, despite the limitations due to his refractory catatonia, the psychoanalyst will continue to telepathically carry out his antisocial plans. Telepathy is the communication of thoughts and ideas to someone by nonsensory means. Dr. Mabuse has telepathic powers that allow him to induce trance states in his victims and manipulate them at his will. Though telepathy is a repeated theme in horror film, including demonic possession films and parapsychological horror, in real life it has not been proven to be real.

Under the Nuremberg Laws, Lang was susceptible to persecution due to his Jewish ancestry, which made him leave Germany for Paris in 1934 where he continued to direct before leaving for Hollywood in 1936. In 1960 he completed Dr. Mabuse's trilogy with *The Thousand Eyes of Dr. Mabuse*. Through the decades other film directors including Jess Franco (1972), Claude Chabrol (1990) and Ansel Faraj (2013) have directed their own versions of the film.

During the early period of Germany's Weimar Republic, on the other side of the Atlantic in the United States a cinema industry was growing in parallel. Plays and film adaptations of the famous novel by Robert Louis Stevenson, *The Strange Case of Dr. Jekyll and Mr. Hyde* (1886), were released only a year after its publication. With the advent of silent films in the United States, several adaptations were released. The first, in 1908, was made by William N. Selig, a film that is now lost. In 1920, Paramount produced a famous adaptation starring the then handsome and young actor John Barrymore (paternal grandfather of Drew Barrymore) and Nita Naldi (a popular femme fatale of the silent era). The film, directed by John S. Robertson, started with the following statement: "In each of us two natures are at war – the good and the evil. All our lives the fight goes on between them and in our hands lies the power to choose – what we want most to be we are." Dr. Henry Jekyll is a young physician with a great reputation who spends all his time and energy researching the supernatural and helping the poor. His peers describe him as the Saint Anthony of London. However, Sir George Carew, the father of Jekyll's fiancée Millicent, taunts him after dinner one night, asking him whether by devoting himself to others he could be neglecting himself. Jekyll responds that serving others is a way to develop the self, but Carew replies: "The only way to get rid of a temptation is to yield to it. With your youth, you should live – as I have lived. I have memories. What will you have at my age?" After the conversation, Jekyll begins to explore the natural duality of good and evil and conceives the idea of developing a potion that can turn him into an evil creature that he calls Edward Hyde. Another potion can take him back to the good Henry Jekyll. Under Mr. Hyde's identity, the protagonist starts to visit the night dance halls, opium dens and bars to satisfy his most primitive desires. In one of these bars he encounters Gina, an Italian woman who is accompanying a man who is under the effect of some drug and believes himself to be covered by red ants. Hyde takes Gina home to live with him.

Initially, Jekyll enjoys transforming at night into his alter ego, but the plan does not go as expected. Every time he transforms into Hyde it gets more difficult to go back to Jekyll, and he becomes more evil even when he is Henry Jekyll. Gradually it becomes more difficult for him to separate good from evil, and his fiancée begins to notice that there's something wrong with her lover. One day, Sir George Carew is walking in the street and happens to see Mr. Hyde kicking and stepping on a small boy. He is surprised when he sees Hyde giving a check signed by Jekyll to compensate the boy's father. Carew goes to Jekyll's house asking for an explanation. In view of Jekyll's inability to offer a clear excuse, he states that he won't allow a marriage with his daughter until further clarification is provided. Jekyll's anger immediately turns him spontaneously into Hyde, who then beats Carew to death and flees. Once the situation is out of control, Jekyll can turn into Hyde at any moment. In one scene he goes to bed and sees a huge ghost tarantula that turns him into Hyde against his will. The doctor, conflicted by his misdeeds, decides to remain locked in his house. Seeing that there is no solution to his problems, he decides to commit suicide by poison. When Millicent goes to visit him, she finds an agonizing Hyde that, after dying, turns into Henry Jekyll.

The storyline can be approached from the views of Sigmund Freud's model of the mind. In 1905, Freud proposed a topographical model in which the mind would be divided between the conscious (those thoughts within our awareness), the preconscious (thoughts that could be retrieved from memory) and the unconscious (unaware primitive wishes and thoughts that were often repressed). Complementary to the topographical model, sometime later he developed a structural model. According to this model, the mind or "psychic apparatus" comprised three functional entities: the ego, the superego and the id. The id operated at an unconscious level satisfying our primitive instincts, which often were unacceptable to our consciousness and therefore were repressed to the unconscious mind. The ego would modulate the instinctual drives in a more socially acceptable way and the superego would ensure moral and societal values.

The Strange Case of Dr. Jekyll and Mr. Hyde is the story of a man who represses his most primitive aggressive and sexual impulses to the unconscious mind. However, the visit to the dance hall with his friends would unlock and bring these impulses to a semiconscious awareness. Still conflicted and obsessed with the good, he creates an alter ego with the help of a potion that turns him into a different person. Under Edward Hyde's identity everything is possible. He is evil and looks evil too, and is capable of anything to satisfy his primary needs. When he transforms back to Jekyll, there is no remorse since there are no consequences; Hyde did it, not Jekyll. The case of Henry Jekyll and Edward Hyde has been referred to in the literature as an example of split personality, or double or multiple personality, now called dissociative identity disorder. In these clinical scenarios, a person is unable to integrate some immoral or unacceptable behaviors within the self. An inability of the ego to integrate the id with the superego causes a repression of the instincts led by the id. After a failed attempt to repress one's desires, the id will gain control over the superego and satisfy the most primitive impulses (usually involving erotic fantasies, substance abuse, and aggression). In extreme situations, if these behaviors continue to be unacceptable, all memories of it can be repressed. The person will therefore become apparently unaware of what they have done. This dissociative identity disorder has been long proposed as a psychological explanation for *The Strange Case of Dr. Jekyll and Mr. Hyde*.

Nevertheless this case may be a little different than other cases of dissociative identity disorder. Henry Jekyll seems aware of his unacceptable desires and consciously chooses to take the potion in order to become Hyde and do as he wants. In forensic settings often individuals take a substance such as alcohol or drugs prior to committing a crime. In the United States it is very hard to make a case of insanity defense in these circumstances, especially if the person took the substance purposely in order to be able to commit the crime, which is the case here with Henry Jekyll. In addition, as derived from the film, Jekyll remembers what he did when he was Hyde. In that case, malingering (a conscious behavior, fabricating or exaggerating the symptoms of a disorder for a secondary gain) rather than dissociative identity disorder may be a more likely explanation. Jekyll understands perfectly the consequences of taking the potion and despite that he chooses to do so. Becoming Edward Hyde will not therefore exempt him from guilt.

Robert Louis Stevenson had a conflictive relationship with his father who discouraged him from writing. He was also a chronically ill child with significant breathing problems. That did not stop him from traveling all over the world, something that encouraged him to also become a popular travel writer. During one of his stays in Bournemouth to benefit from fresh air, he wrote his most famous book. The novel explores the duality of good and evil, which reflects the double morality in the Victorian era. He wrote the story in less than a week, something that has made historians speculate whether he was taking cocaine or ergots at the time.

Dr. Jekyll and Mr. Hyde could be seen as a reflection of Robert Louis Stevenson's own inner conflict between right and wrong. The writer grew up an eccentric and strange-looking child; his family was conservative and religious. He decided to grow his hair long, became an atheist and against his family advice he traveled the world despite being afflicted with a chronic respiratory condition that put him on the edge between life and death on more than one occasion. He fell in love and married a divorced woman ten years his senior from Indiana who had three children. Nonetheless, she became the love of his life, and helped him rebuild the deteriorated relationship with his family. In a more speculative manner, Dr. Jekyll and Mr. Hyde could be the result of a cathartic release of Stevenson's own inner conflict between right and wrong.

In 1925, Warner Bros. started to add sound to their movies. Since most theaters in the United States could just afford a piano player, they used a phonograph to record a full orchestra for their films. A couple of years later they released *The Jazz Singer* with synchronized dialogue sequences, and with six songs performed by the protagonist and famous jazz singer Al Jolson. This led to the ascendancy of sound films and the beginning of the end of the silent era.

CHAPTER 3

Vampires

HISTORICALLY, A VAMPIRE OR an undead was a being that was neither dead nor alive and fed from living humans' flesh or blood. One of the first known episodes of vampire hysteria in a population took place in the village of Meduegna, Serbia. At the beginning of the eighteenth century Meduegna, like other cities in Serbia and Bosnia, was ruled by the Austrian Empire. Serbia had previously been under Turkish Ottoman rule and during this time was devastated by the Austrian–Ottoman wars. During this period, Serbian people lived poorly. Austrians often offered free land to militiamen as an exchange for helping control the area and to prevent a Turkish invasion. One of the earliest documented cases of vampirism was Petar Blagojevich who died in 1725 in the village of Kisilova. His death was followed by nine others within a few days. Soon, some people claimed that Blagojevich had attacked them at night. Even Blagojevich's wife said that he had come to visit to ask her for his shoes. As a result of the increasing tension, the local authorities agreed to the exhumation the body. The examiners found signs of vampirism such as growing hair and nails and absence of decomposition. Fearing more deaths, the locals urged for Blagojevich's body to be staked through the heart and burned.

Another alleged case of vampirism was that of Arnold Paole who before his return to Meduegna claimed to have suffered a vampire attack in Greece. Paole went back to Meduegna in 1727 and continued with his life but died after breaking his neck due to a fall from a hay wagon. Soon after his death rumor spread that he had been seen in different areas. This led to local panic (as this man had claimed to have been bitten by a vampire). Forty days after his death, officers from Belgrade summoned locals to assist with the exhumation of Paole's body. To the surprise of the witnesses there, the body was still fresh and there was fresh blood in the mouth. The body was declared a vampire and staked publicly. Legend says that after being staked the undead Paole screamed and bled profusely. To prevent further vampire activity, his body was beheaded and burned.

More than a hundred years later, in 1892, a new incident of vampirism took place in Rhode Island in the United States. Due to an epidemic of tuberculosis, several members of the Brown family had perished within a short period of time. Fearing that a vampire was causing the deaths, the dead bodies of the already deceased family members were exhumed and it was found that the body of Mercy, one of the daughters, did not show signs of decomposition (the body, however, had been buried in a vault above ground in near freezing temperatures). To prevent further calamity, the family extracted Mercy's heart and mixed it with water. This mixture was offered to Mercy's brother Edwin, who was already sick, as a remedy for his infection. Edwin, however, died soon after, likely from tuberculosis.

Vampire stories probably provided an answer to locals in small villages for several unexplained deaths that occurred within a relatively short period of time. Europeans suffered several devastating plagues in history, including the Black Death, which resulted in an intense fear of new plagues and devastation. Vampire theories offered an explanation with a solution – to find the undead and stake their body – with the hope of stopping the deaths. Medically, these cases of vampirism were likely related to small plagues or contaminated food and water.

Some scholars have explained vampirism as due to pellagra (a niacin vitamin deficiency) in Eastern Europe after the introduction of corn as the main diet. Corn lacks niacin and the lack of this vitamin can cause dermatitis, diarrhea, cognitive problems and bleeding gums. Another disease that has been linked to historical accounts of vampirism is rabies, an infection transmitted by the bites of bats – another icon of vampirism – dogs or wild animals.

The case of the Brown family of Rhode Island received significant media attention. It is believed that Bram Stoker became familiar with Mercy's story as it has some parallels with the character of Lucy in his novel *Dracula* (1897). Bram Stoker was born in Dublin and after graduating from Trinity College married Florence Balcombe (whose former suitor was Oscar Wilde) and moved to London to work as an assistant to actor Henry Irving who owned the Lyceum Theatre. Stoker used to spend the summers in Whitby, a city that served as the inspiration for his horror novel, and while there he read a book on Romanian history at the local library. He probably read about Vlad III, also known as the Impaler (1431–1477), a Romanian hero who led the wars against the Turks to protect Romanians from an Ottoman invasion. Vlad III got his name Dracula (son of Dracul) from his father Vlad II, who had become a member of the Order of the Dragon (Dracul) in Hungary. The order had been founded by Sigismund of Luxemburg (then king of Hungary) to protect Christians from a Muslim Ottoman invasion. Vlad III became notorious in Western Europe for his cruelty towards his enemies; he killed and impaled thousands of them. As a result, Vlad III became an icon of terror in the arts. For instance, a 1499 German woodcut by Markus Ayrer depicts Vlad III feasting among the impaled bodies of his enemies. A fifteenth-century painting of Pontius Pilate judging Jesus at the National Gallery of Slovenia uses the iconography of Vlad III to represent Pilate. Stoker's novel was initially titled *The Dead Undead* and the creature was named Count Wampyr; however, a few weeks before its publication he changed the name of the novel and the main character to Count Dracula. The actor Henry Irving is thought to have served as inspiration for Stoker to develop the attractive and well-mannered aristocratic Count Dracula.

The novel was published initially in 1897 and though it received positive reviews, it only became successful after German director F.W. Murnau adapted it for screen. Together with Enrico Dieckmann, Albin Grau had founded the production company Prana Film in Germany in 1921. Grau had an interest in the occult and alchemy and had become interested in vampires after meeting a Serbian farmer who told him that his father had been attacked by an undead while fighting for Germany in World War I. Grau and Dieckmann agreed to produce a film based on Stoker's novel. For that, they hired Henrick Galeen, who had been the writer of Wegener's *The Golem: How He Came into the World*, and F.W. Murnau for the direction of the film. Grau remained in charge of the production, costumes and design, which made him accountable for the Count's eccentric and tenebrous looks. In *Nosferatu*, the Count does not possess the aristocratic charm of Stoker's Dracula; instead he is a bat-like anthropomorphic figure with long pointed ears and nails, more congruent with the folkloric accounts of vampires. Galeen also had the idea of depicting a Count surrounded by rats. The little mammals were responsible for the plagues and were an allegory of the calamities of Continental Europe.

The film, released in 1922, was set in the city of Wismar, and the old Saltzspeicher building of Lübeck served as Nosferatu's house. Due to copyright limitations, different names were used in the script. In the film, estate agent Mr. Knock sends one of his employees, Thomas Hutter from Wisbourg in Germany, to Transylvania somewhere near the Carpathian Mountains to close a real estate deal with Count Orlok. Once he arrives in the region he sleeps in an inn where the locals try to prevent him from going to the Count's house. Hutter ignores the advice and hires a coachman but he declines to carry him any further after nightfall. Hutter then continues his way on foot until a new black coach picks him up to transport him to the Count of Orlok's castle. Once there, Orlok offers him dinner and closes the real estate deal. The Count becomes especially interested in buying the house after seeing a picture of Hutter's beautiful fiancée Ellen. The next morning, Hutter wakes up with fresh bites in his neck. That morning he rereads a vampire book he had borrowed from the inn and begins to suspect Orlok of being Nosferatu (The Bird of Death). Hutter cowers in his room as midnight approaches, but Orlok enters, his true nature revealed, and Hutter hides under the bedcovers and falls unconscious. Later he is able to escape through the window but

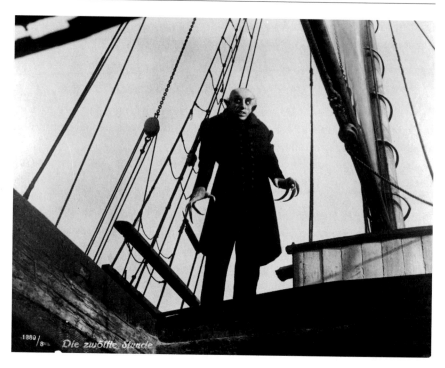

FIGURE 3.1 Nosferatu, the Bird of Death, Brings the Plague to City of Wisbourg (*Nosferatu*)

hits his head, falling unconscious. He awakes in a hospital and hurries home. In the meantime Mr. Knock (Hutter's boss) has become insane and is confined in an asylum. He now has an obsession with eating insects and spiders to absorb their life force. He somehow can feel Orlok's presence in the city. When Orlok arrives in Wisbourg the entire crew of the boat is dead, and Orlok's last victim, the captain, has steered the boat while tied to the rudder. Local physicians conclude that the city is dealing with a new plague, which causes chaos and panic in town. Orlok has a special talent for accessing locked places as a shadow figure. During the night he enters Ellen's room through the window, bites her while sleeping, but becomes distracted with Ellen's beauty and pure heart to the point of forgetting about the upcoming sunrise. When the rooster crows, Orlok vanishes with the first rays of sunlight that enter through the window. In an homage to Stoker's original unpublished ending of his novel, the film's final scene shows Orlok's ruined castle in the Carpathian Mountains, symbolizing the end of his reign of terror.

The film premiered on March 4, 1922 at the Berlin Zoological Garden and received positive reviews. However, Stoker's wife received an anonymous letter informing her about the copyright infringement of her deceased husband's novel. She then sued Prana Film and ordered the destruction of all the copies made. Some copies survived and the film soon achieved cult status, and today it is believed by many film scholars to be the greatest vampire film ever made.

For Werner Herzog, *Nosferatu* was the greatest German film ever made. As a result he decided to remake the film in 1979 in an attempt to link the earlier German Expressionist films of the Weimar Republic with the New German cinema. Herzog's film *Nosferatu: Phantom der Nacht* (The Phantom of the Night), later retitled *Nosferatu the Vampyre*, stays loyal to the original story of Nosferatu. Klaus Kinski stars as Count Dracula. The chaos in the city upon Hacker's arrival in Wisbourg is reminiscent of the town of Rottweil's Narrensprung or Fools' Procession.

In addition to being more consistent with the traditional folkloric accounts of vampirism, *Nosferatu* is a story about fear of death; it reflects the panic that enveloped Europe with the arrival of unexplained deaths caused by plagues. At times when a scientific explanation was not possible, locals would look for a religious explanation (a punishment from God for bad behavior) and occasionally darker explanations with possibly quicker solutions such as black magic or vampirism.

The first Dracula of Hollywood was influenced by the iconography of the Broadway version's famous stage play. Resulting from the success of the play, in 1931, Universal Pictures released Hollywood's first *Dracula*. Tod Browning was appointed to direct the film. For the cinematography German Expressionist artist Karl Freund (*The Golem* and *Metropolis*) was hired. Initially the plan was to cast actor Lon Chaney who became popular after his role in *The Phantom of the Opera* (1925), but he died during production of *Dracula* and instead Bela Lugosi, who starred in the Broadway production, was cast. Rumor has it that Hungarian émigré Lugosi barely spoke English at the time. For Roger Ebert, there is a clear parallel between Dracula's isolation in his Gothic castle and Lugosi's isolation as an immigrant in the United States.

In Browning's *Dracula*, Renfield is a solicitor who travels to Transylvania to discuss leasing Carfax Abbey in London for Count Dracula. The Count, a vampire, hypnotizes him and takes him by ship to London. Once they arrive in the city, everyone but Renfield, who is now a crazed slave of the Count, is dead. Renfield is soon transferred to an asylum near Carfax Abbey under the care of Dr. Seward. In an almost comic manner, Renfield is depicted as a psychotic person obsessed with eating live insects and spiders. Dracula is portrayed as a mysterious and attractive aristocrat with a seductive accent. Dracula meets Renfield's psychiatrist Dr. Seward in a theater and is introduced to his daughter Mina and her fiancé John Harker, along with her friend Lucy. That night Dracula visits Lucy's room and sucks her blood. Lucy dies the next morning. In the meantime, Seward's supervisor Professor Van Helsing analyzes Renfield's blood and discovers that he has been the victim of vampirism, and Dracula visits Mina's room in the middle of the night and bites her, which makes her fall ill. Suspicion arises when Van Helsing realizes that the Count is not reflected in a mirror during a regular visit. Dracula uses his hypnotic powers to manipulate Mina's caretaker so that he can kidnap her and take her to Carfax Abbey with him. Van Helsing and Harker, knowing that the Count would probably be asleep at sunrise, enter the Abbey and stake him. This releases Mina from his hypnotic influence.

As opposed to the original conception of Dracula, in Browning's film, Dracula is a more marketable handsome man from high society with a seductive accent. The film is the first to include the three brides of Dracula. Faithful to the scenography of the stage play, Dracula can transform into a huge flying bat. Hypnosis as a skill to manipulate victims is revisited here. Similar to Caligari and Mabuse, Browning's Dracula uses hypnosis to carry out his plans.

At the time *Dracula* was made, it was common in Hollywood to make a foreign version of the same film using the same studios and set during the night. While Browning and Freund were filming with Lugosi and the rest of the cast during the day, at night George Melford directed the Spanish version of the same film starring Spaniard Carlos Villarías as Conde Drácula.

In clinical psychiatry, Renfield syndrome refers to a psychiatric disorder characterized by an individual's obsession with drinking blood. A person who suffers Renfield syndrome could hypothetically go through several stages: firstly by drinking one's own blood, secondly by eating insects that are alive (like Stoker's Renfield) and finally by drinking others' blood from blood banks or living persons. A reference to this strange blood thirst syndrome is made in the classic Krafft-Ebing's psychiatric textbook *Psychopathia Sexualis* (1886). In current nosological terminology, Renfield probably could be understood as someone who becomes psychotic (a state of impairment of ability to discern reality) with the delusion that he needs to eat live insects and absorb their force. As delusions are illogical beliefs that don't respond to argumentative reasoning, a person with Renfield syndrome will continue to do so despite no evidence of benefit from it. The character of Renfield gradually deteriorates and resembles a man with schizophrenia (a disorder characterized by two or more psychotic symptoms for a prolonged period: delusions, hallucinations, disorganized thinking, or negative symptoms).

In 1958, British company Hammer Productions produced *Dracula* (released in the US as *Horror of Dracula*), directed by Terence Fisher. In this classic, Christopher Lee portrays for first time the character for which he became famous. In this version, Jonathan Harker is hired by the Count as the new librarian in the castle. During his stay there, Dracula's bride attempts to bite him before the Count stops her at the very last moment. The next morning Harker finds he has been bitten and realizes that both Dracula and the bride are vampires. He stakes and kills the vampire woman who suddenly becomes a very old woman, suggesting her real age and her state as vampire. Before he can stake Dracula, sunset arrives and Dracula turns Harker into a vampire. Sensing there's something wrong with his friend, Dr. Van Helsing goes to Dracula's castle in Klausenburg and finds that Harker is now a vampire. He stakes and kills him and returns to Harker's home to inform his family about the suspected vampiric outbreak. Before this, Dracula, seeking revenge for the death of his bride, finds and kills Lucy – in this film, Harker's fiancée – by sucking her blood. Lucy wakes up a few days later as a vampire. Van Helsing convinces Lucy's brother Arthur, Mina's husband, to open Lucy's grave during the day and is astonished to find she does not have any sign of decomposition. Realizing that she has become a vampire, Van Helsing stakes her. At the same time, Dracula has bitten Mina, who is now under his influence and is taken to his castle in an attempt to turn her into his next bride. Arthur and Van Helsing go to the castle to prevent Dracula from burying her alive. As they arrive Van Helsing and Dracula begin to fight. When the first rays of sun appear in the castle room, Van Helsing opens the curtains and using the repelling effect of a crucifix improvised with two candles, he gradually presses Dracula into the light, which turns him into dust.

In these later versions of *Dracula*, the erotic connection with vampirism is more established. Obviously, Count Dracula is now depicted as a middle-aged, wealthy dapper beau who seduces with his talk. From a more psychoanalytic perspective, several fantasies are narrated in Dracula's story. First, we must take into consideration that Stoker's *Dracula* was written in the Victorian era, a time of sexual repression. Sigmund Freud himself claimed that dreaming about vampires was related to repressed sexual impulses.

In Stoker's story, John Harker goes to the Count's castle and is kidnapped by three of Dracula's beautiful and sexy brides. (Among the most common fantasies in men is to engage in sex with more than one female partner.) As a counterpart, the attractive Count travels to London and bites the defenseless Lucy and Mina while they sleep at night (perhaps a female sexual fantasy).

The vampire's erotic bites could represent a regression to an oral stage of development. According to Freudian psychoanalysis, in normal sexual development, during the first year of life, the baby's erogenous zone is the mouth. During this phase, the baby suckles the breast of the mother and places other objects in the mouth as a source of pleasure. In adult life, under stress, we all can engage in activities that relate to an oral fixation in order to alleviate stress. For example, smoking a cigarette, chewing gum, biting a pencil, or even eating cookies as a response to a stressful situation are examples of oral fixation behaviors that can help relieve stress. In sexual intercourse or when two individuals feel a strong sexual or romantic attraction the first impulse usually involves kissing on the mouth, or kissing several parts of the partner's body before penetration. In fact, oral sex usually precedes penetration. From that perspective, the viewer may experience a cathartic pleasure when watching a vampire biting the neck of his victim.

From a psychoanalytic perspective, vampires are allegories of unacceptable sexual desires or impulses that, in conflict with a superego (due to conservative societal values), are not integrated within the ego and are repressed in the unconscious. As we can see in the *Dracula* films, the vampire acts on the erotic impulses of the id, and becomes repressed again with the aid of religious symbols such as crucifixes, holy water and holy hosts, objects that symbolize superego-related values. In a more speculative manner, the stake used to kill a vampire can be seen as a penetrating phallic symbol.

Considered one of the most influential directors of all time, in part due to his masterpiece *The Passion of Joan of Arc* (1928), Carl Theodore Dreyer grew up in foster homes in Denmark. It would not be hard to guess that his upbringing impacted his films, which are characterized by recurrent deep psychological themes. Dreyer spent most of his childhood with a foster family in a liberal home. *Vampyr* (1932) was Dreyer's first sound film. The French–German production is centered on the fictional character of Allan Gray. In the opening scene Gray arrives at an inn in the village of Courtempierre, France. There he meets Gisele and Leone, the daughters of the Lord of the Manor. They appear to have some kind of sickness. At the inn Gray finds a book about the history of vampires and discovers that many years before, in the same village, there was an epidemic that took the lives of eleven people. Though doctors provided a scientific explanation, rumor had it that the real cause of the epidemic was the vampire of Marguerite Chopin, a woman who lived an evil life and died without remorse. Gray also learns that there was a doctor who sold his soul to the Devil and was helping a vampire. At that moment Gray understands that Gisele and Leone are victims of vampirism and that their physician is a servant of Marguerite Chopin.

Dreyer's story is the most faithful to the historical accounts of vampirism in Europe. Symbolically, the film can be approached from the realms of the Electra complex. Contrary to the belief of Sigmund Freud that both women and men competed for the love of their mother in the Oedipus complex, Carl Jung proposed that little girls, as opposed to boys, compete with their mothers for the love of their fathers during the phallic stage of psychosexual development. In *Vampyr*, two girls who live with their father fall sick under the curse of an evil woman. Perhaps their sickness is the result of a neurotic manifestation in an attempt to compete for their father's attention. Once Gray appears in the picture as a new male, providing a potential sexual pairing, the conflict can be resolved successfully.

As with Oedipus, the character of Electra was central to one of Sophocles tragedies. In Sophocles' tale, King Agamemnon of Mycenae sacrifices his own daughter Iphigenia as commanded by the gods. When he returns from the Trojan War with a new concubine, Clytemnestra, Agamemnon's wife and mother of Iphigenia, kills both of them in revenge. Many years later, Electra – another daughter of the couple – will kill her own mother with the help of her brother Orestes to revenge her father's death.

In one scene of *Vampyr*, Gray has a vision of being buried alive. The lack of knowledge about catalepsy, catatonia, narcolepsy and other sleep disorders meant that during the Victorian era it was suspected that a person suffering one of these rare conditions could potentially have been buried alive. Edgar Allan Poe reflected this type of fear in one his short stories "The Premature Burial." This fear, described in the literature as taphephobia, led to the construction of safety coffins, which included air tubes and the connection of the limbs to an above-ground safety bell, and to houses of the dead, where dead bodies were taken for observation until they showed signs of putrefaction. In 2010's *Buried*, Ryan Reynolds plays Paul Conroy, who works as an American truck driver during the Iraq War in 2006. Conroy wakes up in pitch darkness and slowly realizes that he is trapped inside a wooden coffin, buried alive. He has been left with a cellphone that allows him to make calls and contact the outside world. However, he has a limited amount of battery life and air to orchestrate his own rescue plan. This claustrophobic film reflects the potential panic that a person could face if buried alive.

The second novel of famous horror novelist Stephen King was *Salem's Lot* (1975), the title being an abbreviation of the town where the storyline takes place, Jerusalem's Lot, in Maine (King's birth state and the setting for many of his works). The first film adaptation came four years later. The story starts with the return of successful writer Ben Mears to his hometown, Salem's Lot, Maine. Ben comes with the intention of spending some time writing a novel about the town's haunted old Marsten House. Ben still vividly remembers seeing a ghost inside the house when he was ten years old and believes that the manor is an evil house that attracts evil men since many tragic events have taken place there. However, Ben discovers the house has just been rented to the macabre-looking Richard Straker, an antique dealer whose partner Kurt Barlow is often mentioned but is always absent.

During his stay in Salem's Lot, Ben also meets the lovely teacher Susan Norton and soon begins a love affair with her. However, Susan was seeing Ned Tibbets who is not ready to give up on her. Susan had a failed attempt to leave the small town and live in New York City. Now Ben, a famous writer, represents an opportunity to follow her dream one more time. In contrast, if she stays with Ned Tibbets, a local plumber in town, it will mean the acceptance of her current life. While Susan's dad seems to like Ben, Mom does not approve of him. In fact, Susan makes a statement that her mom only likes Ned Tibbets. Perhaps she fears that Ben will finish the book, go back to New York and break her daughter's heart. Or perhaps Mom is not satisfied with her current routine life in the small town and is unconsciously jealous of her daughter who now has the opportunity to have a different life.

In the meantime, Straker kidnaps a young boy named Ralphie Glick in the forest to offer him to the vampiric Barlow. Ralphie becomes a vampire and in the middle of the night he goes back home to claim his brother Danny who he bites in the neck. As a result, Danny also becomes a vampire and hypnotizes the local gravedigger in order to bite him. Soon a vampire plague starts in town. Danny also claims the body of his school friend Mark at night. However, Mark is a horror film fan who knows how to recognize and repel vampires. In the middle of the chaos people start to leave the town, scared of the plague. Barlow kills both Mark's parents during an altercation with the local priest. Barlow also kidnaps Susan. Ben goes with Mark to rescue his lover and discovers that Barlow sleeps in a coffin surrounded by the rest of the people in town who have turned into vampires. Ben is able to stake Barlow in the heart, killing him, and then sets Marsten House on fire.

In a different scene, Ben and Mark are in Guatemala two years later, where they receive the unexpected visit of Susan as a vampire. Ben attempts to kiss her and in grief kills his own lover. Then Ben and Mark leave to continue wandering around the world escaping from the surviving vampires of Salem's Lot.

Kurt Barlow's vampire features are strongly influenced by the aesthetic of Count Orlok in *Nosferatu*. Both have a repulsive appearance, long nails and ears, and visible teeth. When the box containing Barlow arrives from Europe there are also rats – an allegory of the plague – around it. Consistent with historical accounts of vampirism, the vampires can only get into the house and bite their victims if they are invited by the host, and they sleep at night, do not tolerate daylight and are repelled by Catholic symbols like crosses. As in Browning's *Dracula*, vampires use hypnosis to control their victims prior to biting them. However, the new vampires are more like the traditional European accounts of the undead. They seem to be living dead, looking more like zombies than being seductive and attractive. Through biting, they transmit their infection and spread the disease of vampirism. This is also an allegory of rabies, a disease that threatened Europe since the origin of civilization and spread to the United States in the eighteenth century.

In one scene in *Salem's Lot*, the local priest confronts Barlow with a cross; this refers to the previously mentioned battle of the id (the vampire) versus the superego (the priest). Marsten House is very similar to *Psycho's* Bates House and both are decorated with stuffed animals (regular props in horror films after Hitchcock's classic). For King this is one of his favorite books that to an extent reflects the reality of small towns nowadays in America. Similar to the accounts narrated in *Salem's Lot*, today small towns and rural life in the United States are in danger of disappearing.

1974's British film *Vampyres* by Spanish director José Ramón Larraz takes the mythical vampiric male sexual fantasy to an extreme. In his film, a couple of striking lesbian vampire women abduct and seduce passing men on the road, invite them to their house and make them participate in their orgies of blood and sex. In contrast, Joel Schumacher's *The Lost Boys* (1987) offers the puritan teenage version of a vampire movie. In the film, Mike and his younger brother Sam move with their recently divorced mother Lucy from Arizona to their grandfather's home in Santa Carla in California. The town's boardwalk is full of flyers of missing people. Mike begins to hang out with one of the local gangs after falling for Star, the girlfriend of the gang's leader David. Mike meets two vampire hunters, the Frog brothers, at a book store. Against Star's advice, Mike drinks from a bottle of wine David offers and the following day he begins to feel blood thirst. David persuades Mike to kill people to drink their blood but Mike is trying to resist the urges of his new nature. With the help of the Frog brothers, Sam is able to stop the gang from recruiting Mike, but we discover that the true vampire leader is their mom's new boyfriend.

The Lost Boys reflects the changes from childhood to adolescence. Mike and Sam seem to have had a good and close fraternal relationship. It is likely they relied on each other to get over their parents' divorce and now they move together from a quiet city in Arizona to a new town with a lot of perceived threats. Mike is now an older adolescent who falls in love with Star. Sam probably resents that he is losing his brother and is on his own. Furthermore, Mom has found a new boyfriend, so Sam loses his two main supports. While Mom is distracted dealing with her own problems, Sam is witness to how his older brother is changing after hanging out with the wrong people. In real life this could well have been a scenario in which gang members are introducing Mike to drug use. In fact the bottle of wine in the film well reflects a moment in which the adolescent would be initiated into drugs after feeling the gang's pressure. Mike is initially hesitant but he surrenders. Sam is the only one who realizes the dangers that his brother has been exposed to and will do whatever he can to save him. Once his brother is saved, Sam can focus in the other threat, Mom's new boyfriend. Sam probably feels it might be too soon for him to see his mother with a new man. Most likely, he still hopes that his parents will eventually get back together. That is why it is important to prevent his mom from finding new love, at least for now.

Another important teenage vampire movie of the 1980s is *Fright Night*. The film was unexpectedly a box office success and became the second highest grossing horror film of 1985 after *A Nightmare on Elm Street 2: Freddy's Revenge*. In this vampire film, Charley Brewster is a teenage horror film fan with a lovely girlfriend called Amy. Charley is also a fan of a TV presenter called Peter Vincent, a former vampire hunter. Charley doesn't appear to be delusional but he witnesses his new neighbor Jerry Dandridge and his partner Billy with a dead body. Charley begins to connect the new crimes announced on TV with his neighbor and watches from his window as Jerry is about to bite one of his victims. The next day, the same person is announced missing on TV. Charley tries to talk to his mom, his friend Evil Ed, his girlfriend and the police about what is happening but no one seems to believe him. Finally he asks his hero Peter Vincent, the TV vampire hunter, who does not believe him either. Charley's mom invites Jerry to the house, something that according to the vampire rules would allow him to enter the house freely. That night

Jerry breaks into the house and threatens Charley. In the interim Amy and Evil Ed ask Peter Vincent for his help to talk to the neighbor and see if he can show to Charley that he in fact is not a vampire. During the visit, Peter discovers Jerry is a vampire because he is not reflected in a mirror, but he does not say anything. That night, Jerry turns Evil Ed and Amy into vampires. Amy has an astonishing resemblance to Jerry's lost love and his plan is to keep her for himself. With Peter's help, Charley will attempt to stop the vampire's malevolent plans.

Jerry is an older attractive man. He seduces Charley's mom to get in and hypnotizes Charley's girlfriend. Jerry is seductive, dresses well and has his own house. It would be very hard for Charley to compete with him. In general, women and especially younger girls tend to feel attracted to older men. As portrayed here, during adolescence, males tend to be in a situation of inferiority when competing with older men for sex partners, something that can be very frustrating. Nonetheless, Amy seems to be a nice girl with feelings for Charley. The moment in which Jerry bites Amy is charged with sexual connotations. Moreover, Jerry and Billy seem to live in a homosexual relationship. Once again, the relationship between vampirism and free sexuality is patent within the film.

Francis Ford Coppola directed his version, *Bram Stoker's Dracula*, in 1992. Here Dracula's depiction is influenced by the iconography of Vlad III, the Impaler. He has long hair and a mustache that make him resemble a noble man from Renaissance Transylvania. The first scene of the film is set in the fifteenth century. Elisabeta, Vlad Dracula's fiancée, commits suicide in despair after receiving a false report that her lover has died in combat with the Turks. Once he returns home from the battle, enraged by his fiancée's fate, Dracula renounces God and in a chapel he stabs a stone cross then drinks the blood that pours from it, thus becoming the prince of darkness. Coppola's *Dracula* is a love story, in which, after acting against the world for centuries, he falls in love again after meeting Mina in 1897. Though still conflicted, his love for Mina challenges his evil actions and makes him reconnect with the good. Once defeated, he asks Mina to help him find peace. She stabs him through the heart then decapitates him, breaking the curse he had fallen under some 500 years earlier. Dracula then dies a good person and goes to heaven with his fiancée Elisabeta. Coppola's *Dracula* is more a story of becoming a better person after finding love. This idea goes more in the direction of the clear Christian iconography and messages we see in Hollywood's last two decades. The film, however, attempts to connect with the past and pays homage to silent films. In one scene, we can see an old room for cinema projecting one of the first moving pictures ever made: *Arrival Train* (1895) by the Lumière brothers.

The story of Dracula has often been interpreted in psychoanalytic circles as an example of an Oedipal victory. So Dracula is depicted as a powerful figure who attempts to compete with Jonathan Harker for the love of Mina. In this case a triadic relationship is not possible and after being killed with a stake – a phallic symbol – Harker will continue his monogamous love with his fiancée. Menstruation, blood and bodily fluids are all psychodynamic elements that connect sexuality to vampirism.

Interview with the Vampire is a 1994 film directed by Neil Jordan based on the novel by Anne Rice who also wrote the script. In this film, Lestat and Louis are two homosexual vampires in New Orleans who share a female child vampire, Claudia. Due to irreconcilable differences, Louis takes Claudia with him to Paris where they find Armand who tries to seduce Louis to stay with him at a theater with other vampires. In this story, we see vampires who have feelings and attempt to fight their nature in order to be good, trying to feed themselves on rats to avoid taking human lives.

Based on Marvel comics, *Blade* (1998) is about a superhero vampire of the same name, half human, half vampire; he kills vampires to protect other humans. *30 Days of Night* (2007) portrays the least sexual image of vampires. Here, vampires are animalistic monsters with unusual strength who try to kill everyone for the mere purpose of feeding themselves in a small town in Alaska during wintertime.

Among the more recent vampire films, perhaps the most successful and praised by critics is Tomas Alfredson's *Let the One Right In* (2008). Set in a suburb of Stockholm, twelve-year-old Oskar is a lonely only child who lives with his mother and is bullied in school. His father is an alcoholic who lives in the countryside. His life changes after becoming friends with Eli, a child vampire who becomes Oskar's best and only friend. She gives him the courage to confront the bullies. Eli lives with an older man, Hakan, who kills and drains the blood of random people to supply Eli with the blood she needs. When Oskar discovers Eli is a vampire he struggles with the conflict of her nature and his love for her.

In the film Hakan is a pedophile who is in love with Eli and dedicates his life to her after he turns into a vampire; he won't repress his desires for Eli and will attempt to rape her. Though not revealed in the movie, according to the novel Eli turns out to be a eunuch who was sadistically castrated by a vampire nobleman centuries earlier. Since ancient times, royal and noble people had the practice of castrating men at an early age to prevent the development of sexual hormonal changes. These eunuchs had an important role in high society where they functioned as servants, sexual partners, singers, advisers, or guardians of harems. In psychoanalysis, castration anxiety refers to a concept developed by Sigmund Freud in relation to the phallic stage of sexual development (between three and five years of age). According to Freud, during this phase the child competes with the father for the love of his mother. While a boy child may experience castration anxiety fearing that his father will castrate him to win such a competition, a girl may experience penis envy, feeling that her father has already castrated her and consequently losing the competition for her mother. This symbolic competition is referred to as the Oedipus complex (inspired by the ancient Greek story of King Oedipus who unknowingly killed his father and married his mother). In a good resolution of the Oedipus complex, the boy or the girl will understand that both his or her parents can love each other at the time that they love him or her. In that case, the child will learn how to master triadic relationships. A lack of resolution of the Oedipus complex will result in an inability to master triadic relationships. In real life, we commonly encounter situations that challenge our ability to master triadic relationships. We often display feelings of jealousy when people that we care about show appreciation for others. This can be especially challenging in romantic relationships, where exclusivity becomes an essential value and to an extent gives us the dyadic relationship security that allows us to function in society. Immature people often have an inability to function in triadic relationships and demand constant attention and exclusivity from everyone they encounter. This is an unrealistic demand that when not met will lead them to maladaptive behaviors that interfere with their ability to function in society.

CHAPTER 4

Monsters

A MONSTER IS AN imaginary creature that is usually large, frightening or ugly. Among all monsters, perhaps Frankenstein has become the most popular in cinema.

In 1780, Luigi Galvani was a professor at the Academy of Science at the University of Bologna where he taught anatomy by human dissection to the medical students, participated actively in debates and published a paper every year at the academy. That year, he became interested in animal electricity after finding that he could make the muscles of a frog leg contract and kick when stimulated with electric current in the sciatic nerve. This discovery implied that muscle contraction was the result of electricity carried in a liquid rather than air as it had been thought earlier in the scientific community. Animal electricity (later coined "galvanism" in homage to its discoverer) gave birth to electrophysiology, a science that still is a major field of research, especially in neuroscience and psychiatry.

The experiments of Luigi Galvani became very popular across Europe and attracted the attention of Mary Godwin and many other intellectuals of the time. Mary was still very young when she met one of her father's political followers, poet Percy Shelley. Soon they started a romantic relationship and together traveled through Europe. After Percy Shelley's wife died of suicide, Mary and Percy got married. In a trip to Geneva, Switzerland with friends Lord Byron and John Polidori, a challenge was made to see who could create the best horror story. Mary, while still a teenager, wrote a novel in 1818 titled *Frankenstein; or, The Modern Prometheus*. According to Greek mythology, Prometheus was a Titan and a trickster who gave the human race the gift of fire and the skill of metalwork, thus disobeying the will of the gods. He was therefore punished by Zeus who chained him to a rock and ensured that an eagle would come every day to eat his liver. Fortunately for him, many years later, the hero Heracles would kill the eagle with one of his arrows and free the ailing Titan from eternal suffering. In other traditions, Prometheus was also credited with the creation of the first man from clay, which was likely the

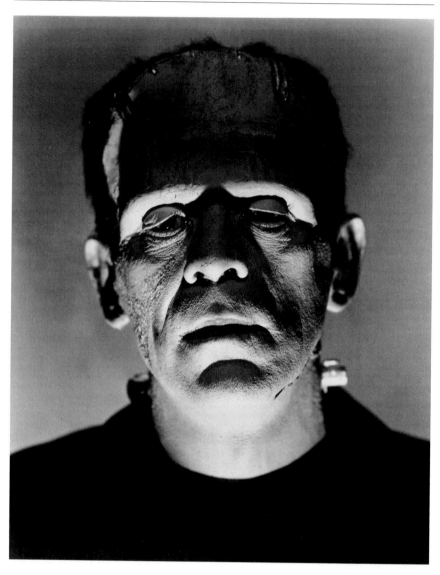

FIGURE 4.1 The Monster Created by Victor Frankenstein (*Frankenstein*)
© NBCUniversal

reason that Mary Shelley called her fictional character Victor Frankenstein, the modern Prometheus. Due to its success, Shelley's book soon became a stage play and one of the first horror films ever made.

In 1910, Edison Studios in New York produced the sixteen-minute kinetoscopic film *Frankenstein*, directed by James Searle Dawley. In the short film, the young student Frankenstein becomes obsessed with the mystery of life, and with some chemicals in a vat he is able to create a human being that forms from a skeleton. The creature, however, turns out to be an aberrant being, as a result of Frankenstein's impure and evil ideas. The monster shows up unexpectedly during Frankenstein's own wedding, but, overwhelmed by the love of the couple, the monsters vanishes.

After the success of Browning's *Dracula*, Universal Pictures released a series of monster horror films. British director James Whale was commissioned for the Hollywood version of Shelley's novel. Boris Karloff was cast to play the monster. Initially the role was offered to star Bela Lugosi but he left the project due to disagreements about the development of the character's personality.

In the Universal version, *Frankenstein* (1931), Henry Frankenstein and his hunchbacked assistant, Fritz, steal bodies from cemeteries and other sources in an attempt to create a new life by experimenting with electricity. In an anatomy lecture, at the Goldstadt Medical College, the professor Dr. Waldman explains how the brain from a normal person is different from the brain of a criminal based on the scarcity of convolutions in the frontal lobe. These anatomical features, according to the doctor, explain the criminal's history of violence and brutality; in other words, it is the anatomy of the criminal mind. After the students leave the class, Fritz steals the normal brain but drops the container, breaking the glass, after hearing a noise and instead takes the abnormal brain. Frankenstein and his assistant spend all day in his castle obsessed with his experiments without allowing any visitors. Worried, Frankenstein's fiancée Elizabeth and friend Victor Moritz call Henry's professor, Dr. Waldman, to express their concerns about Henry. The professor tells them that Henry had gradually changed during the time that he was becoming obsessed with human life. He had abandoned his medical studies and was no longer a student there. Upon Elizabeth's request, Dr. Waldman agrees to visit Henry Frankenstein in his castle. In a different scene, Henry and Fritz are surprised in their castle by the visit of Elizabeth, Victor and Dr. Waldman in the middle of an electrical experiment where they are attempting to animate a body he has created with lightning from a storm. Initially hesitant, Henry agrees to share with them the specifics of his experiments. He tells Dr. Waldman that as he learned a lot from him about ultraviolet light as the highest color of the spectrum he is now about to prove that he was wrong. After that he uses lightning to pass all the electricity through the body and when the creature's hands begin to move, Henry makes his now famous announcement: "It's alive!"

Dr. Waldman warns Henry about the danger of his experiments, which Henry ignores in grandiose fashion. Dr. Waldman informs Henry that the brain Fritz stole in the school belonged to a criminal and alerts him that he has created a monster. He encourages him to think of his father and fiancée. Henry claims that in a few days his experiments will be proven right and will change the course of science forever. He says he does not care about his father because his father never believed in anyone. The conversation is interrupted by the monster's first few steps. Then, the famous iconic image of the huge flat-headed creature (Boris Karloff), with a screw in either side of the neck to facilitate the electrical conductivity, follows. The creature is a giant being with the mind of a child who still has to learn about coordination and gross and fine motor skills. He is also unable to talk. Fearing the whole experiment went wrong, Fritz tries to scare the monster away with a torch. Disappointed with his results, Henry and Dr. Waldman hide the monster in a room and leave. They inject him with a tranquilizer, which makes him fall unconscious. Henry becomes disinterested in his creation and leaves the castle to organize his wedding with Elizabeth. Meanwhile, Waldman stays at the castle with the sedated monster. He soon realizes that the creature needs increasing doses of sedatives to stay calm, and he decides to destroy it. However, at that time, the monster wakes up and strangles the professor. Right after, he flees and encounters a little girl by the lake. He starts playing with her by throwing flowers on the water. When they run out of flowers, the monster throws the girl into the water, thinking she may float too, and then he leaves. Henry and Elizabeth continue to make their wedding arrangements but on the wedding day, Elizabeth has a premonition that something bad is going to happen. Soon, the monster breaks into the house and scares the bride. Next the father of the little girl the monster had thrown into the water shows up in town with the dead body of his daughter. The people of Goldstadt immediately accuse the monster and start a search. Henry is separated from the group and is discovered by the monster, which attacks him. The monster knocks Henry unconscious and carries him off to an old mill. The peasants find the monster has climbed to the top, dragging Henry with him. The monster hurls the scientist to the ground but the vanes of the windmill break his fall, saving his life. The villagers set the mill on fire with their torches and the monster dies entrapped within.

In Whale's *Frankenstein* there are several elements that relate to maladaptive narcissism. In the first place, Henry Frankenstein's castle is among the most phallic structures seen in Hollywood films. Henry shows narcissistic traits. He drops out of medical school, interested in what he believes are bigger matters. In a grandiose statement he says the world will admire his creation that will change the way we understand life and believes that his ability to create life will elevate him to a God-like level. Henry tells Dr. Waldman that everyone will be mesmerized by his work and legacy. Waldman advises him to think about his father and his fiancée. Henry replies that his father did not believe in anybody. From a psychodynamic point of view this is the most important statement in the film in relation to pathological narcissism. Heinz Kohut, a major contributor in the field of narcissism, believed that all psychopathology in adults could be derived from inadequate attention and nurturing from their caregivers. A failure to provide the child's needs results in a psychological tragedy such that grandiosity and lack of empathy will be subsequent survival defenses. While grandiosity will help people forget their inferiority complex, a lack of empathy will keep the disconnection between the false grandiose perception of the self and the real vulnerable and anxious one. Henry is therefore portrayed as a grandiose person who does not seem to care about others' concerns about him. His statement about his father supports this theory.

In contrast, the monster portrayed by Boris Karloff is an intellectually challenged man. His brain is less convoluted and belonged to a criminal. His flat head suggests lack of brain matter for the size of his skull. From a developmental perspective, the monster has just been born and is attempting to learn the same things any infant would. He slowly learns how to coordinate his extremities in order to walk. He innocently and unwillingly kills the little girl as at his stage of development he does not yet understand the abstract concept that while some objects can float, others don't. Furthermore, he is unable to talk. From a psychiatric viewpoint an argument for autism could be built based on his language impairment; however, the monster is craving human relationships and is frustrated by his inability to do so and by the rejection he experiences. As a result he tries to take revenge and kill his father and creator. The monster has just been born and is still learning; for his early age he might actually be performing at a developmentally appropriate level. However, knowing the kind of brain that was implanted in him, we should not have great expectations about his potential.

When the monster takes his first steps he becomes combative and obstinate. The monster is first secured in a room and the professor later injects an intramuscular sedative in him to control his agitation. In this scene, a clear reference to the psychiatric methods of restraints at the time is made.

The monster as portrayed here has clear parallels with Paul Wegener's golem in *The Golem*. In both films a creature is made out of dead material. In fact Prometheus, more consistent with the golem narrative, had created the first man out of clay. In contrast, Frankenstein or the modern Prometheus makes a man out of human parts of other men and uses his knowledge of the most updated scientific advances – galvanism – to create life. Both Frankenstein's creature and the golem are huge anthropomorphic figures that could potentially follow the orders of their creators. In both films, one of the most remarkable scenes is when the monster encounters and interacts with an innocent young girl.

Even before *Dracula*, in 1957 Hammer Productions released *The Curse of Frankenstein*. In the film, directed by Terence Fisher, Peter Cushing portrays the mad scientist Victor Frankenstein, and multifaceted Christopher Lee was cast to play the monster. The film is narrated by an imprisoned Victor Frankenstein who awaits his execution by guillotine. The story starts with Victor being forced to live alone after becoming an orphan and hiring Paul Krempe to tutor him. Gradually Victor becomes interested in resuscitation with the use of alchemy and electricity. Krempe is initially as enthusiastic as Victor but he drops out after learning about the ethically questionable ideas Victor proposes. Victor is collecting body parts in order to create a perfect being. Victor's narcissism switches to an antisocial level. In Machiavellian fashion, he kills a respected professor by pushing him downstairs while distracting him with a copy of Rembrandt's *The Anatomy Lesson of Dr. Nicolaes Tulp*. After the professor's body is buried, Frankenstein intends to raid his tomb and extract his brain. Krempe surprises him and attempts to stop him. In the struggle the glass containing the brain is broken, possibly adding more damage to the brain to that already suffered by falling down the stairs. In the meantime, Victor's fiancée Elizabeth arrives to stay with them. Victor continues his experiments and when he is about to abandon the project due to poor results, a lightning strike animates the body and the creature begins to breathe. The monster tries to strangle his creator, but Krempe intrudes and helps his friend. The monster is locked up, but it escapes. Victor and Krempe start a search for the monster in the forest and Krempe shoots him in the head, killing the creature. After that, Victor's mistress, Justine, begins to blackmail him to make him marry her instead and threatens to tell the authorities about his unethical experiments. Victor revives the creature to make him kill his mistress. Anything is possible as soon as his energy is directed towards his own benefit. The film initially portrays an orphaned young Victor who is given a lot of responsibility, but according to psychiatric theory, a lack of paternal care could certainly contribute to his antisocial lack of empathy.

The Curse of Frankenstein centers on the figure of the mad scientist. The mad scientist archetype as depicted by Dr. Caligari and Dr. Mabuse is even more clearly seen in this film version of the novel than in the Hollywood one. Victor has no problem with killing in order to achieve his goals and shows no remorse for the consequences of his actions, nor empathy for his victims. This is also clear in the scene where he humiliates and taunts his mistress when she tells him of her feelings for him. In *The Curse of Frankenstein*, the villain is not the creature but the creator.

Kenneth Branagh directed *Mary Shelley's Frankenstein* in 1994, which is the most faithful film version of the original narrative. Robert De Niro was cast to play the creature and Helena Bonham Carter the bride. Here, Victor Frankenstein (played by Branagh), frustrated by the loss of his mother, goes to medical school with the intention of surpassing conventional science in an attempt to resuscitate the dead and prevent humans from dealing with grief and loss. His models are Paracelsus and other great scientists who did not necessarily play by the rules. In this film, the creature is intelligent and has memories and feelings. He confronts his creator, asking him whether he had thought about the consequences of his actions. In this film the monster echoes the eternal questions of human existence: "What of my soul? Do I have one?" – a question that the creator is unable to answer. Branagh's Frankenstein tale is a story of love and isolation; the creature craves company in order to fulfill his life, as happiness is not possible if not shared or witnessed by another human being. He asks his creator for a female companion in exchange for disappearing and moves to the North Pole, the only place where there are no humans. Branagh's tale is also one of loss, grief and death anxiety.

Inspired by the Universal Pictures Frankenstein movie and other classic horror sagas of early Hollywood, Tim Burton directed the animated horror comedy *Frankenweenie* in 2012, a remake of his own 1984 original short film. Burton's *Frankenweenie* revisits the idea of grief and loss from a child's perspective. For children, often the first time in their lives this occurs is when facing the death of their first dog or other pet. Burton claimed he wrote the first film as a cathartic reflection to deal with the loss of his own first dog. In the film, Victor Frankenstein is a young boy who loves science and film-making and spends most of the time with his canine best friend Sparky. Frankenstein's eccentric science teacher Mr. Rzykruski introduces the children to Luigi Galvani's frog leg experiment. After Sparky dies after being run over by a car, the young Victor resuscitates him with the use of the principles of animal electricity. At first, Victor is happy enjoying the return of his best friend but he is discovered by his classmate Edgar who agrees to keep the secret as soon as he helps him reanimate his two dead goldfish. However, the experiment does not turn out the way expected and the dead goldfish become invisible piranha-like dangerous fish. Edgar reports Victor and their foreign science professor Mr. Rzykruski gets blamed and fired after he stands up for himself with his memorable and wonderful speech to the parents of New Holland:

"Ladies and gentlemen. I think the confusion here is that you are all very ignorant. Is that right word, 'ignorant'? I mean stupid, primitive, unenlightened. You do not understand science, so you are afraid of it. Like a dog is afraid of thunder or balloons. To you, science is magic and witchcraft because you have such small minds. I cannot make your heads bigger, but your children's heads, I can take them and crack them open. This is what I try to do, to get at their brains!"

Before he leaves the school, Mr. Rzykruski advises Victor that a scientific experiment will have a good or bad outcome depending on the heart you put in it and its purpose. Now, Victor's classmates, with the only ambition of competing to win the science class award, use animal electricity to reanimate sea monkeys, and other dead pets. Elsa Van Helsing's cat Mr. Whiskers, a cat with a special talent for predicting bad events through the shape of its feces, is electrocuted by lightning, turning it into a cat-vampire. Sparky dies again while trying to rescue Victor from Mr. Whiskers at the burning windmill. Moved by Sparky's heroic actions, the people of New Holland resuscitate Sparky one more time with the electricity in their car batteries so that Victor can see his friend again.

Another popular Universal Pictures monster is the werewolf. Lycanthropy is the belief that a human can metamorphose into an animal, usually a wolf. Since the time of ancient Greece and Rome, lycanthropy reports have appeared in literature. During the early modern period, werewolvery was a practice associated with witchcraft. Alleged witches were therefore subject to accusations of turning a normal person into a werewolf. One of the first historical accounts of werewolverism was the case of Peter Stubbe in Rhineland, Germany. Also known as the werewolf of Bedburg, Stubbe, a farmer, was arrested in 1589 and under the coercion of torture he confessed to having used a magic belt given by the Devil that allowed him to transform himself into a huge wolf. He admitted that in this werewolf state he had devoured children and pregnant women. He also confessed to having intercourse with a succubus or female demon sent by the Devil. As a result, Stubbe and his daughter were sentenced to death as Stubbe had also been accused of having an incestuous relationship with her. On October 31 (coincidentally Halloween in Western folkloric culture), Stubbe suffered one of the most brutal executions in history: he was put in a breaking wheel, having all his limbs beaten and broken, and then he was decapitated and burnt. It is believed that Stubbe could have been a wealthy new Protestant in the area and therefore his execution could have been used politically and religiously to prevent other Germans from converting to Protestantism.

Another famous case of werewolf hysteria took place in Gascony, France in 1603. Fourteen-year-old Jean Grenier was accused by three witnesses of turning into a wolf to eat cattle and drink their blood. When thirteen-year-old Marguerite Poirier revealed that she had been attacked by a huge werewolf, a number of people identified Grenier as the alleged aggressor. He was therefore arrested and taken to the high court, where he confessed to all the charges. The child even accused his father Pierre Grenier of sorcery and wolverism. When interrogated, the father was believed to be a simple rustic man who had no idea about his son's alleged activities. Indeed Jean Grenier had run away from home after his father beat him and had been wandering around stealing food and trying to survive the best way he could. Due to his youth and extreme ignorance, Jean was not sentenced to death but instead imprisoned in the Franciscan friary of Saint Michael the Archangel.

Accusations of witchcraft, werewolverism and black magic were popular in central Europe during the Renaissance. An engraving of a huge werewolf, running away from a house with a baby in its mouth after mutilating a number of bodies, by Lucas Cranach the Elder, can today be seen at The Metropolitan Museum of Art in New York.

Nicknamed "The Wolfman" (Der Wolffsman), Sergei Pankejeff was a patient of Sigmund Freud in Vienna in 1910. The analyst published the case later in 1918. According to Freud, the analysis centered on a dream the patient had as a young child. In the dream he would wake up in the middle of the night, open the window and see six or seven white wolves that threatened his life. The patient would wake up horrified by the idea of being eaten by the wolves and it would take him a while to get back to sleep. Both the patient and the analyst agreed that the dream was an unconscious representation of having seen his parents having sex "doggy" style. The ability to consciously discuss that with the analyst led to a cathartic release and alleviation of the patient's neurosis. This case helped Sigmund Freud to both support the validity of psychoanalysis and develop his psychosexual development theory. With this theory, Freud addressed sexuality as the major drive and acknowledged sexuality in children since the moment of their birth: oral (up to one year), anal (one to three years), phallic (three to five years), latent (six to eleven years), and genital (adolescence and sexual maturity).

In the film arena, after the relatively poor reception of *Werewolf of London* in 1935, a new werewolf movie was released by Universal in 1941, *The Wolf Man*. Lon Chaney Jr. was cast to play the werewolf. The laborious make-up used to turn the man into the beast is today regarded as a significant milestone in the history of make-up in film. Curt Siodmak wrote the screenplay and the now legendary poem that citizens in the film narrated every time someone talked about werewolves:

> *Even a man who is pure in heart*
> *And says his prayers by night*
> *May become a wolf when the wolfbane blooms*
> *And the autumn moon is bright*

In the film, Larry Talbot goes back home after the mysterious death of his brother in a small town in Wales. There he falls for a local girl, Gwen, who tells him about the werewolf superstition in town. One night Gwen is attacked by a werewolf and Larry successfully saves her, but not without first being bitten by the beast. A local gypsy woman, Maleva, informs Larry that her son Bela while in the state of being a werewolf was the one who bit him and now he too will become a werewolf. Maleva's prophecy turns out to be right and Larry, as a wolfman, begins to commit murders at night that he barely remembers the following morning. One night, the werewolf is killed with a silver cane by Larry's father who contemplates with horror how the beast turns into his son.

The narrative of *The Wolf Man* has evident similarities with Stevenson's *The Strange Case of Dr. Jekyll and Mr. Hyde*. Scholars believe that was probably the main reason for its initial unsuccessful reception. In both, a benevolent person turns into a malevolent one to commit murder. The repressed impulses are materialized in the animal or evil side of the same person. Nevertheless, in *The Wolf Man*, in contrast to Jekyll, Larry did not intend to become a wolfman and kill people. For Larry, this was more of the misfortune of a random attack by Bela, the werewolf son of the gypsy woman. However, under the beast state he won't be able to repress his unconscious impulses, will murder, and will approach the woman he loves, something he was unable to do as a normal human. When Larry comes back to human form in the mornings, he barely remembers what he has done the night before. Once again, here we see the inability to integrate the id-related behaviors within the ego, a mechanism that provides the basis for dissociative identity disorder. A gypsy fortune teller advises Larry about his new nature. Curt Siodmak successfully incorporates the old folkloric belief that vampires are sensitive to silver into his werewolf story and links witchcraft to wolverism with Maleva's character. Likely inspired by the ancient Greek narrative of King Oedipus, *The Wolf Man* is the story of a man cursed by the fate of his inner demons who is unknowingly killed by his estranged father at the moment he is attacking the woman he loves. Here, instead, the father kills the son before the sexual fantasy takes place. The movie was remade in 2010, with Benicio Del Toro playing the beast.

An American Werewolf in London (1981) is a British horror comedy written and directed by John Landis. It tells the story of David and Jack, two American friends who are attacked by a werewolf while traveling in England. Jack dies during the attack but David survives and becomes a wolfman. Jack's spirit remains on Earth to inform his friend that he has turned into a wolfman and must kill himself before he commits more crimes. David struggles to believe his friend and with killing himself. In real life, many people often say that if they suffer a severe impairing stroke, or terminal disease, they would rather kill themselves than go to treatment. However, in general these statements are said out of overwhelming anxiety. Most people end up getting treatment and take any chance to go on living. In the case of David the situation is even more complicated, as his disease is affecting third parties. The will to live is almost biologically programmed and, as portrayed in the film, even when our death or sacrifice could potentially save the lives of other people we will struggle to the end with our deep and inherent will to survive.

Also during the 80s, Stephen King published a short story on lycanthropy. A film based on his story called *Silver Bullet* was released in 1985. The tale concerns the struggles of Marty, a child with a physical disability, and his dysfunctional family. Although Marty is wheelchair bound he seems to be well adjusted. He has friends, and has as much of a normal life as he can get. He is also well liked by people in town. His sister Jane resents that he gets more attention from his mother. His mother Nan, however, seems to struggle with having a disabled son, as she foresees Marty's limitations in the future. Marty's father is not in the picture. The male figure in the house is Uncle Red who gives Marty a lot of attention and joy but has severe alcohol addiction. As a result Nan doubts whether he is a good influence in Marty's life. When a series of unexplained murders occurs in the quiet town, the residents meet to decide how to hunt down the killer. Many end up dead and their efforts to find the assailant don't take them anywhere. After getting a new motorbike from his uncle, Marty encounters a werewolf one night at the time he is using some fireworks on a bridge in the forest, and the pieces begin to come together. Along with his sister and his uncle, Marty begins a mission to capture the werewolf, which turns out to be the town priest.

Psychoanalytically, the priest represents the two poles of the mind, the superego (the priest) and the id (the werewolf), one for the day and the other for the night. However, when discovered, the evil starts to flourish within the day. The priest shows no remorse and makes every effort to not get caught. Perhaps he has an antisocial personality as well. Nonetheless the most interest centers on the character of Marty. In general children with medical disabilities have normal peer interactions and don't necessarily have any more social problems than other children. However, this does not apply to children with central nervous system disabilities in which their problem is visually apparent and so they can suffer stigmatization. In these particular cases, stronger support must be offered to prevent future social difficulties with other peers. Marty seems to have a very satisfactory social life. He is a popular kid. In fact his sister resents the lack of attention. While sibling rivalry is common in most families, in cases where there is a disabled or medically ill child, the siblings can resent lack of attention from their parents and extended family. For parents, it can become a real challenge to divide attention in a way that they are providing their sick child the care needed while not neglecting the other siblings' developmentally appropriate needs. In these cases the assistance of extended family or a mental health professional can be helpful.

Clinical lycanthropy refers to a pathological belief that one can turn into an animal form. The kind of animal will vary and is thought to be culturally bound but the wolf is thought to be one of the most common types. Psychodynamically, lycanthropy may be understood as a manifestation of an acceptable sexual or aggressive impulse. Commonly this belief reaches a delusional level and appears in the context of the psychiatric symptomatology of a patient with schizophrenia or other severe affective disorders that can carry an impairment of reality testing, usually implying the need for antipsychotic medication for its treatment. Lycanthropy has also been described in the context of alcohol intoxication, and ecstasy and other psychosis-inducing drugs. In that case, the removal of the offending agent will be the first therapeutic intervention.

The story of a resuscitated mummy became another famous Universal monster. Ancient Egyptians believed that three parts formed the soul: the *ka*, the *ba* and the *akh*. The *ka* would stay in the body and within the confinements of the burial tomb. The *ba* would be able to flee the tomb and go to other places, and the *akh* would go to the underworld for judgment to gain an entrance to the afterlife. Mummification was an important process in an attempt to preserve the body and the *ka*, the part of the soul that could enjoy all the objects and offerings placed in the tomb with the deceased person. Initially mummification was costly and exclusive to pharaohs and very wealthy people but later it became more inexpensive and available to a higher number of people.

A good preservation of the body became important to enjoy the afterlife and the art of mummification became gradually more complex over the centuries following early Egyptian civilization. A normal mummification process included pulling the brain out of the nose using a hook, and after an incision in the left side of the body all the organs were extracted to leave the internal cavities exposed to the air to allow a drying process. The lungs, intestines, stomach and liver were placed in jars and the heart would be replaced back into the body. The inside of the body would be later rinsed with wine and spices and the corpse was covered with salt for seventy days to prevent decomposition. Forty days later the body was filled with linen to give it more volume and human shape and then seventy days later it would be covered with bandage before being placed in a sarcophagus.

After Napoleon's campaigns in Egypt from 1798 to 1801, a series of publications written by scholars who accompanied him was published from 1809 to 1829, called *Description de l'Égypte*. These books focused Western international attention on Egypt and popularized Egyptology. Mummies brought from Egypt were displayed for the enjoyment of visitors in stores, circuses and even private shows where a mummy's bandages were often removed. Products from mummies were also marketed for medical use and to make paints. Scholars have often referred to this mummy fashion as the mummynomania of the nineteenth century. In fact, Mark Twain jokingly stated in a travelogue that mummies were used as fuel for the train from Cairo to Alexandria.

Germany, France, Italy and United States sponsored campaigns to travel to Egypt and learn more about the ancient civilization. In 1922, the tomb of Tutankhamen was found. This discovery gained international acclaim as it was the first unlooted Pharaoh's tomb ever found, permitting important advances in Egyptology studies.

Inspired by the discovery of Tutankhamen's tomb and the Curse of the Pharaohs (a belief that any person, including archeologists, who disturbs the mummy of a Pharaoh could become ill or die), and the success of Dracula and Frankenstein films, producer Carl Laemmle Jr. decided to make an Egyptian-themed horror film with Universal Pictures. John L. Balderston, a journalist who had covered the story of the discovery of Tutankhamen's tomb, was hired to write the script and Karl Freund, who had already participated in the *Dracula* movie, was hired to direct the film. Balderston used the name of the famous ancient architect, physician and philosopher Imhotep to develop the mummy character played by Boris Karloff. In the film, Sir Joseph Whemple and his assistant Ralph Norton have identified the ancient mummy of Imhotep. Legend says that he was mummified alive as a punishment for attempting to resurrect his forbidden lover, Princess Ankhenesamon. Recklessly Ralph reads an ancient life-giving scroll which revives the mummy who escapes into Cairo in search of the contemporary reincarnation of his ancient lover. Years later, Imhotep, disguised as a contemporary Egyptian, helps the two archeologists find the tomb of Princess Ankhenesamon and the mummy and treasures are given to the Cairo Museum. In that context, Imhotep encounters Helen Grosvenor, whom he believes to be the modern reincarnation of his beloved princess. As a result he attempts to kill her with the purpose of mummifying her and resurrecting her to make her his bride. Helen prays to Isis who saves her and turns Imhotep into dust.

Historically Imhotep has been associated with the oldest medical text ever written, the "Edwin Smith papyrus," named after the dealer who bought it in 1862. To date, this papyrus is the first known surgical treatise and consists of forty-eight cases of trauma patients of which the first twenty-seven discuss head injuries. Among them the first descriptions of the meninges and convolutions of the brain are discussed. One of the patients discussed has a head injury affecting the temporal lobe that interferes with his inability to talk, an area later identified as Broca's area and the cortical location for speech. The papyrus is today displayed at the Brooklyn Children's Museum in New York.

William Indick argues that like previous films, the mummy revisits the Oedipal myth in which the "jealous father" (the Pharaoh) punished "the son" (Imhotep) by being buried alive for his forbidden love with "the mother" (Princess Ankhenesamon).

After being reanimated by the scroll read by Ralph, Imhotep flees to modern society in search of the modern reincarnation of his lost loved one. In romantic relationships, it is fairly common to see that after the break-up of a meaningful relationship, a person frequently finds a new lover who resembles their previous lover. The similarities between the past lover and the new lover can be psychological and often physical, in an unconscious attempt to replace the loss of the loved one. Imhotep believes to have found the reincarnation of his former lover, Princess Ankhenesamon, in Helen, a woman who strikingly resembles her physically. According to psychodynamic theory, the original ideal love model would be initiated by the mother. Once emancipated, the son would search for a person with whom he can psychologically reproduce the kind of relationship formed between them and the first caregiver in the search of safety and intimacy.

In contrast, Helen is unaware of Imhotep's inner psychological drives and perceives the mummy as merely a threat to her own life. For most humans, the first call for help in extreme situations that may threaten one's own life is the religious or spiritual call. Consistent with that, Helen prays and Isis, the Egyptian goddess that historically listened to the prayers of the wealthy and aristocrats, successfully saves her from her final fate.

A sea monster is a legendary creature that inhabits the sea. Historically, sailors have reported seeing sea monsters on their voyages. These monsters could often be immensely big and a potential threat to the sailors. Depictions of sea monsters were also used for decoration in maritime cartography. Accounts of sea monsters have been made through the centuries across different places and cultures. Many of the alleged sea monsters may have been dolphins, whales and giant squids and octopuses. According to Greek mythology, Triton was the son of Poseidon and messenger of the sea; he was depicted as a half man–half fish god figure. According to a Polish legend of the sixteenth century, Bishop-fish was a sea monster that was caught and brought before the king. After asking for help from a group of Catholic bishops, he was released and after making the sign of the cross, Bishop-fish disappeared into the sea.

Perhaps the last of the great Universal movie sagas was 1954's *Creature from the Black Lagoon*. Directed by Jack Arnold, the motion picture was one of the first released in 3D. It narrates the story of a geology expedition in the Amazon based on the story and idea that producer William Alland wrote inspired by the legend of a half human–half fish creature in the Amazon River and the traditional fairy tale *Beauty and The Beast*. Likely the story that Alland had heard was the legend of Yacuruna. According to the local indigenous people of the Amazon, Yacuruna was a monster who inhabited the Amazon and could turn into a dolphin with the ability to detect the odor of menstruating woman. Once a woman was located, Yacuruna could turn into a handsome and seductive man to kidnap her and take her to his kingdom underneath the water.

In the Universal film a scientific expedition in the Amazon River is led by Dr. Carl Maia and Dr. David Reed, a well-known ichthyologist, in the search of an ancient fossil. Also in the crew there are the young and beautiful Kay Lawrence, Reed's girlfriend; Captain Lucas; and Dr. Edwin Thompson. After failing to find the fossil they decide to go down the river and see if they have better luck. In the meantime the Gill-man creature discovers Kay's existence when she is swimming in the water, and he begins to voyeuristically examine her while swimming alongside. After a few failed attempts in which different crewmembers are killed, the Gill-man kidnaps Kay and takes her to his kingdom in the depths of the river. David is able to dive down to the kingdom and rescue his lover, and once the rest of search group arrives they start to try to kill the creature, but a merciful David stops them from shooting him. The agonizing creature manages to go back to the river and disappear.

Among all the Universal monster films, *Creature from the Black Lagoon* is the one that best represents Sigmund Freud's first model of the mind. Beneath the big lagoon is the unconscious and the small boat represents the conscious life. What happens on the surface of the water is the preconscious mind or the in between. The monster, or the unacceptable impulses of the id, is initially at the bottom of the lagoon hidden and apparently imperceptible among the algae. Seeing the beautiful girl in her bathing suit swimming on the surface is a significant stimulus that begins to alter the balance of the ego. The monster gradually begins to swim towards the surface in the direction towards consciousness. Initially ambivalent about allowing his impulses to reign, the creature is hesitant to take the lady with him and she has enough time to return to the boat. However, as the Gill-man's impulses become harder to repress, the creature at some point crosses the surface of the water and mounts the boat, "becoming fully conscious," to kidnap the young lady and take her to his kingdom. Dr. Reed and the rest of the crew are the superego. Until that moment, Kay had been with them for the entire trip and no one had made a pass at her, not even an innocent gesture. Immediately after the creature kidnaps the beautiful lady, the superego reacts and rescues her. The unacceptable behavior of the creature is brutally punished by the rest of the crew who start shooting at the poor creature without mercy. Finally, in an effort at integration with the ego, Dr. Reed stops the rest of the crew from continuing to shoot the Gill-man in an unconscious attempt to keep the id alive.

CHAPTER 5

Aliens from Outer Space and the Paranoid Horror

AFTER THE FALL OF Berlin to the Allied forces in 1945, two superpowers emerged. Once standing together against Nazi Germany, the United States of America (USA) and the Union of Soviet Socialist Republics (USSR) soon began to have significant political, economic and social differences. The tension concerning these two countries between 1947 and 1991 has been known historically as the Cold War, as direct active fighting between the two foes never took place. Nevertheless, they tested their forces by supporting and taking opposite sides in regional wars such as Korea, Vietnam and Afghanistan and to a lesser extent in Latin America and Africa. The Cold War took place at a militaristic, scientific and economic level. Both countries had nuclear weapons, and while the Russians were the first to travel outside planet Earth, the Americans were the first to step on the moon. The Americans exported a capitalistic economic model while the Soviets proposed a Marxist–Leninist one.

As a result of this tension, so-called communist paranoia flourished in the United States during the 1950s, a time in which Wisconsin Republican Senator Joseph McCarthy declared that there were many Soviet spies in the country. Witch-hunt hysteria grew against anyone suspected of sympathy for communism. It is estimated that hundreds of people were imprisoned and up to 10,000 lost their jobs due to suspicion of communist activity. Hollywood became a high-profile target for McCarthyism. Charlie Chaplin, Luis Buñuel, Arthur Miller and Orson Welles were examples of targets of this type of persecution, forming part of the so-called Hollywood Blacklist.

With the disasters of World War II, fear of a new nuclear war and the potential devastation caused the growth of a new paranoia in American society. Helping to relieve this anxiety was a popular interest in science fiction which resulted in a new golden wave of horror-science fiction films and literature.

A number of films with themes about invaders guided by a harm principle saw light in theaters. Aliens from outer space, giant ants or monsters that threatened human existence became the new villains. These threats have been referred to by scholars as a metaphor for the fear of Soviet defeat or invasion and the uncertainty about possible annihilation as a result of a new nuclear war.

In 1951, four years after the beginning of the Cold War, producer Julian Blaustein took the lead in the making of a film that characterized this new era of atomic power: *The Day the Earth Stood Still*. Edmund North was hired to write a script based on Harry Bates's short story "Farewell to the Master." One of Frank Lloyd Wright's most notable works, the Johnson Wax Headquarters (1939) served as inspiration for the interior of the spacecraft.

Directed by Robert Wise, the film narrates the story of an alien named Klaatu who arrives on a spacecraft in Washington DC at a time of significant international political tension. Despite announcing his coming in peace as soon as he leaves the flying saucer, he is immediately shot by a reckless soldier. Right after, a robot named Gort leaves the spacecraft and begins to neutralize the weapons until Klaatu asks him to stop. Klaatu is then taken to a hospital where is treated by doctors who are surprised by his rapid healing as well as his apparent youth and physical health despite being seventy-eight years old. Klaatu appears to come from a far more advanced civilization. He states that he came from his planet with the intention to deliver to all representatives of all nations an important message. However, the authorities tell him that to do such a thing would be impossible in the Cold War political climate. Instead they put him into custody of the state. Later, Klaatu manages to escape to stay in a boarding house where he meets Helen and her son Bobby. Klaatu babysits Bobby who shows him around the city and takes him to the Arlington National Cemetery to visit the tomb of his father who died in combat during World War II. Klaatu and Bobby agree on how meaningless all wars are and imagine a world without them. After visiting the Lincoln Memorial, Klaatu shows admiration for the historic president and asks Bobby to take him to the greatest living person. Bobby takes him to Professor Barnhardt. After they meet, Klaatu advises the professor that other planets will eliminate the Earth if this wave of violence continues. In a demonstration of power, Klaatu is able to black out all electricity on Earth at the time that he reveals his secrets to Helen. Authorities begin an exhaustive search for the alien and shoot him to death. Gort rescues the body and takes him to the spacecraft where he is resuscitated. Right before leaving on the spacecraft he gives a final message to all terrestrials, stating that the universe grows smaller every day, and the threat of aggression by any group, anywhere, can no longer be tolerated. Men are free to act with responsibility and live in peace, but if they continue this aggression, an army of robots will destroy the Earth. Klaatu gives terrestrials a choice: join us and live in peace, or pursue your present course and face obliteration.

The parallels between Klaatu and Jesus Christ are evident. Klaatu presents himself among lay people as Mr. Carpenter, alluding to the trade that Jesus began prior to starting his spiritual journey. Both befriend children and are morally and intellectually superior to any other human being. The two seem to have special superpowers, talents or gifts. Both are just men, killed for preaching a true message that could save the world from self-destruction, a message that will only be listened to by imperfect humans and repeated following their resurrection. In that sense, Klaatu is the Messiah of the 1950s Cold War. The story of a just man who is betrayed and killed for preaching his ideas is a recurrent theme in Hollywood cinema.

Similarly to Wise's film, in Universal Pictures' *K-Pax* (2001), prot (uncapitalized) is an alien from a distant galaxy. Believed to be a delusional person, he is committed to a psychiatric hospital in Manhattan under the care of Dr. Powell, who treats him with the antipsychotic drug haloperidol and hypnosis. After several failed attempts prot is finally able to convince his psychiatrist of his true nature and advises him that people from K-Pax, his planet, have discovered that humans are determined to make the same mistakes again and again to eternity.

In contrast to the benevolent approach in *The Day the Earth Stood Still*, that same year Christopher Nyby directed *The Thing from Another World* (1951), which offers the counterpoint to Robert Wise's Messianic version of an alien from outer space. The screenplay was written by Howard Hawks, along with Charles Lederer and Ben Hect. The Thing is an evil alien that instinctively attacks humans and feeds from blood, bodies and organic flesh in order to reproduce in an asexual form. The alien had crashed on Earth in Alaska thousands of years ago. In the current time, the saucer is discovered by a group of scientists and men from the air force, led by Dr. Carrington and Captain Hendry, by detection of residual radioactivity with the use of a Geiger counter. The frozen alien is detected, extracted and taken to their station. As the ice melts, the alien revives and escapes, but not before having his arm severed by the sled dogs, and left on the ice. Dr. Carrington discovers the alien needs blood to survive after incubating seedlings from the alien seedpods. They soon discover that the alien in fact had been feeding from a sled dog and two of the scientists that are found dead in the greenhouse. After failing to enter the station to attack the rest of the crew, the alien cuts off the heating fuel cable with the intention of freezing them to death. In a final attempt to survive, the crew is able to electrocute and kill The Thing with an electric fly trap.

With the advances of nuclear fission science, which led to the discovery of nuclear weapons and the bombing of Hiroshima and Nagasaki, the film has been viewed as a critique of how the use of science can represent a threat to human life. Dr. Carrington is a man who knowingly puts his entire crew at risk with his obsession to understand the underpinnings of the alien's biology, an example of reckless science that, as with nuclear science, could have had devastating results. In contrast to the Jesus-like alien Klaatu, The Thing is a horrendous figure – a tall bald megacephalic with green skin and with spikes in his knuckles and fingertips. The Thing is aggressive and threatens human existence, killing people or dogs (man's best friend) to use their blood and reproduce asexually. Its final goal would probably be to control humans and use them for food, a theme that will be later revisited in other science fiction films such as *The Matrix* (1999). While the character of Klaatu is inspired by Jesus, The Thing is inspired by the Devil.

Legendary horror film director John Carpenter became a big fan of Howard Hawks' classic and in 1982 produced a remake of the film. Carpenter's *The Thing* was made during the end of the Cold War. Though Carpenter wrote the music of many of his films, in this case he hired Ennio Morricone who wrote a magnificent soundtrack that contributed to the fearful atmosphere of the film. Carpenter combines the spirit of the classic film – an alien guided by a harm principle for unclear purposes – with elements of the then popular body horror. The monster here goes for the most part undetected, taking the form of a sled dog, or a crew member, increasing the sense of paranoia within the group: anyone can be the monster. MacReady, the main character played by Kurt Russell, concocts a method for the detection of the monster. He burns the blood of each of the crew members, knowing that the alien's blood will not tolerate the burning fire. In this version, the monster also feeds from human blood. Blair, the scientist of the mission, informs the rest of the crew that if the alien escapes the entire human species could be assimilated in a few years. However, MacReady destroys the monster. In the mythical final scene, another crew member reappears. With the knowledge that they will unavoidably freeze to death they both open a bottle of scotch and drink together. We don't know if they are still humans or not.

Psychiatrically, Carpenter's *The Thing* can be viewed through Capgras syndrome: the delusional belief that a person has been replaced by a looka-like impostor. This syndrome was initially described by Joseph Capgras and his intern Jean Reboul-Lachaux in France in 1923. The delusional symptoms usually happen in the context of dementia, schizophrenia, and other cognitive and psychotic disorders. In Carpenter's film, we never know whether someone is a real person or an identical impostor. This idea had already been explored after Hawks' *The Thing* in two other films: *Invaders from Mars* (1953) and *Invasion of the Body Snatchers* (1956).

The peak of communist paranoia was likely reached with the release of *Invaders from Mars*. The film starts with the boy David MacLean being awakened during a loud thunderstorm to see a flying saucer. He immediately runs to his parents' room to alert them. His father goes and checks outside and returns with a red puncture mark in his neck and a different attitude. David notices how people in town – including his parents – begin to behave strangely; there seems to be something wrong with them. As things get worse, he goes to the police officer and realizes he has a red puncture mark in his hairline too. Estranged by his parents, David is helped by Dr. Pat Blake, a child psychiatrist, who decides to take custody of the boy. With the help of Dr. Kelston, an astronomer, David and Dr. Blake realize that they are suffering an alien invasion from Mars and take action to alert the Pentagon. However, both of them are later sucked underground and kidnapped by two green alien humanoids. They discover that these aliens are implanting mind-controlling devices in the people they abduct to make them sabotage a nuclear project near the town. A fight starts between the US Army and the Martians and in the midst of a huge explosion young David wakes up in his bed again. He goes to his parents' room and apparently everything is normal. The whole film could have just been a boy's nightmare.

Invaders from Mars reflects the popular political message during McCarthyism of the time: communists (like Martians or invaders) are indistinguishable from non-communist subjects, something that increases the community's paranoia even more. Anyone can be a communist and there is no good way to differentiate them so we must be suspicious and we can never be sure. In the realms of psychiatry, again, this idea can be seen through the view of Capgras syndrome. The invaders are identical and indistinguishable from the loved ones they have replaced.

The film also addresses other pertinent aspects in the field of child and adolescent psychiatry, which are reflected in the character of the main protagonist David MacLean. Among the most common childhood fears are fear of thunderstorms, fear of monsters, and fear of being estranged by one's own parents. All of them are represented in the film. In general, most people overcome these fears, though in some cases, these fears, when out of proportion for the developmental level, can hint at clinical signs of future psychopathology. In the case of David, he seems to have a recurrent nightmare about flying saucers arriving in the middle of a thunderstorm. His anxiety is soothed by the reassurance of his parents. In a more traditional psychoanalytic approach we could speculate that David's fears could be the manifestation of a repressed sexual memory (for example, having caught his parents in some kind of sexual activity during one of his unexpected trips to their room in the middle of the night). Finding his parents sleeping and reassuring their love for him would relieve his neurotic anxiety.

In the midst of McCarthy's communist paranoia, Walter Wanger started a production based on Jack Finney's novel *The Body Snatchers*. Wanger initially intended to have Orson Welles involved in an introductory speech but was unsuccessful in casting him. Congruent with the setting of the novel, the film was shot in Mill Valley, California, a few miles north of San Francisco. One of the first characters to appear in the movie is psychiatrist Dr. Hills. Dr. Miles Bennell, a family physician, is the main protagonist of the film. He is brought to psychiatrist Dr. Hills by the local police for evaluation of a possible psychotic outbreak. Dr. Bennell shares his story: after returning from a conference, most of his patients had canceled appointments with him but the few that were still coming reported seeing family members acting strangely. At first he thought a mass hysteria outbreak was happening in town but soon he started to believe there was something more serious occurring, as these people seemed to have lost their human qualities. Bennell and his girlfriend Becky discover that people in town are being replaced by other beings that look physically identical. At some point they find identical lookalike impostors of themselves growing from seedpods in the greenhouse of Bennell's property and realize that they are dealing with an extraterrestrial invasion.

Invasion of the Body Snatchers is an example of McCarthyism communist paranoia. The body snatchers are an allegorical representation of the loss of individuality that communism can carry. The doppelgangers of the characters seem to have no soul. They lack individuality and the group's will prevails. They attempt to convert the protagonist and everyone else into one of them. Once you are one of them you lose your uniqueness and individuality. Though some of the people who participated in the making of the film professed no political intention, the success and popularity of the film is consistent with the preoccupations of society in the 1950s.

Again, from a psychiatric point of view, what happens in the film is congruent with a Capgras delusion. The inverse of Capgras syndrome is Fregoli syndrome, which consists of the sustained belief that the same person is taking different forms and identities. The person suffering a Fregoli delusion would believe, in a paranoid manner, that different people are still the same person manifesting in different forms.

In 1978 Philip Kaufman directed a successful remake of the film for which Donald Sutherland was cast as the main protagonist. His son, Kiefer Sutherland, would later play the role of the doctor in Alex Proyas's film *Dark City* (1998) in which Inspector John Murdoch attempts to discover his identity while being persecuted by a group of extraterrestrial parasites, "The Strangers," who propose a model of collective consciousness and memory in detriment to our individuality. Coincidentally, the same year Robert Rodriguez's *The Faculty* tells the story of a group of teenagers in Ohio who try to survive the invasion of an alien species that adopt the physical appearance of the teachers and the students in their high school.

Existentially, *Invasion of the Body Snatchers* addresses an essential fear: the loss of one's individuality. Are we unique beings? Are we replaceable? This debate often occurs within science with new discoveries in neuroscience and the stress diathesis model of medicine. In this model, our genetically determined genes with the random modifications of the environment shape our brain and with that our mind and personality. These findings challenge our current beliefs about individual freedom and free will and provoke a type of existential anxiety depicted in *Invasion of the Body Snatchers*.

One of the first science fiction color films was the futuristic Metro-Goldwyn-Mayer's *Forbidden Planet* (1956). Directed by Fred Wilcox, the film stars Leslie Nielsen as Commander John Adams, leader of the twenty-third-century expedition starship *C-57D*. After twenty years of travel the troop arrives on the planet Altair IV and is received by Robby the Robot who takes them to encounter Dr. Edward Morbius. The doctor alerts the troop of the danger of an unknown force that killed his entire crew, sparing only his family. Morbius's daughter, Altaira, is a beautiful and naïve young woman who becomes attracted to the newly arrived men. Farman, one of the commanders, makes a pass, something that Adams (who also likes her but represses his desires) finds unacceptable. Altaira, however, shows a preference for Adams against her father's wishes. Soon the troop is threatened by an invisible creature. Adams discovers that the monster is the result of Morbius's unconscious mind manipulating a machine he has created. Through the monster, he is able to carry out his unacceptable impulses driven by the Thanatos or death drives. The film departs from the Oedipus complex to a new scenario, a man's rivalry with his potentially future son-in-law. We know little of Morbius's childhood from the film. However, it is explained that he unconsciously killed his crew years earlier, saving only himself and his wife. Was his wife the only female on that planet? Did he do it to protect her from sexual competitors? Following the death of his wife from natural causes, his young daughter is the only person he has (symbolically the only remnant of his wife). With the arrival of Adams and his commanders, Morbius faces a new threat: if Adams requites Altaira's love, he will face loneliness for the rest of his days. Morbius seems a good-hearted man; his aggressive impulses towards avoiding losing his daughter's company can only manifest through the unconsciously created monster of the id.

As explained earlier, with the Cold War came an intense nuclear paranoia. Both the USA and the USSR had atomic weapons and a hypothetical war between the two superpowers would potentially be the most devastating catastrophe in human history. With the discovery of radioactivity caused by nuclear energy and its potential serious impact on the environment, a fear of the appearance of new mutant species began. *Them!* (1954) is perhaps the first monster movie among a series of films that explore the potential environmental devastation of radioactivity. The film was directed by Gordon Douglas. As a result of nuclear experiments, a new mutant species of giant ants threatens the entire human race. At the beginning of the movie, Sergeant Ben Peterson and his sidekick find a little girl in shock, lost in the desert of New Mexico. Initially confused about what is going on they realize there is a colony of mutant dangerous giant ants nearby. (This scene resembles the beginning of James Cameron's *Aliens*.) Peterson and his team alert the government and report the several victims they find of these aggressive species. The ants have the ability to communicate and their huge mandibles are lethal. With the help of troops sent by the president, they will be able to mitigate the fear and burn the nests of the ants. However, the film concludes that the threat may come back. In a final scene, Dr. Medford reflects on the door that man has left open with the atomic age and our unpredictable future of the paranoid horror genre: the threat can come back any time.

On August 6, 1945, at 8.16 a.m. the atomic bomb "Little Boy" was dropped over the city of Hiroshima, Japan, killing nearly 80,000 people with the direct impact and injuring over 25,000. By the end of that year, another 60,000 people had died from the effects of the bomb. Only one-third of the city's buildings still stood and only twenty out of the 200 doctors in the city were able to continue their profession. After the detonation of the bomb, a wave of X-ray heated air advanced like a fireball faster than the speed of sound, destroying everything within 1.6 miles of the detonation. Many people were vaporized instantly. (One of the victims sitting a few meters away from the epicenter left only a shadow.) Three days later, "The Fat Man," the second atomic bomb, was dropped on Nagasaki, killing nearly 40,000 people.

Though many were injured, fortunately more than two-thirds of the population survived the bombings. Tsutomu Yamaguchi became a survivor of both bombings. While he was from Nagasaki, he was in Hiroshima on a business trip for Mitsubishi Heavy Industries at the time the Little Boy bomb was dropped. Though he suffered several wounds, he went back to Nagasaki and returned to work on August 9, when the Fat Man bomb was dropped. After surviving the two detonations, he put his traumatic experiences behind him and lived to ninety-three years of age.

Nine years after the tragedies of the atomic bombings of Hiroshima and Nagasaki Ishiro Honda's *Gojira* (Godzilla) was released in Japanese theaters. In the film, an ancient creature, a mix of a *Tyrannosaurus rex, Iguanodon* and *Stegosaurus*, is revived in Japan as an effect of the nuclear radiation. The monster surprises the city, breathing fire like a dragon and setting the city on fire while smashing everything it encounters. Dr. Yamane and Dr. Serizawa find the monster's weak spot and save the city from total destruction. However, Dr. Yamane believes that if nuclear energy tests continue, another Gojira will be awakened.

Producer Tomoyuki Tanaka found inspiration from the atomic bomb, feeling that Gojira represents Mother Nature taking revenge for humans creating nuclear energy. The film was very successful, in part due to a probable catharsis in the audience, who were still dealing with the devastation that the bombs had brought. Gojira, like the atomic bomb, is a threat that arrives unexpectedly, destroying the buildings and setting the city on fire in a very short time.

In 2014, Warner Bros produced *Godzilla*. In this version of the film, a monster called MUTO (massive unidentified terrestrial object) lands in Hawaii, destroying a submarine and terrifying everyone. In a new twist, Godzilla engages MUTO and kills him, somehow saving the human race. While MUTO is a dangerous monster, Godzilla in this film is charming. The audience here does not want Godzilla to die. Once Godzilla disappears into the sea, the audience gets a sense of a Hollywood happy ending. Metaphorically, Godzilla could be seen as the American monster while MUTO seems to be the Japanese monster. Director Gareth Edwards' film portrays Godzilla as a necessary evil to prevent what could be even worse: MUTO. This portrait would certainly be more consistent with an American view of the facts of World War II.

In 1958 Irvin Yeaworth cast Steve McQueen, then twenty-seven, in his film debut, *The Blob*. As a result of a meteorite, a gelatinous pink substance grows bigger and bigger as it swallows living people. With the help of his girlfriend, Steve Andrews (McQueen) stops the new threat. As with *Invaders from Mars* and *Invasion of the Body Snatchers*, in *The Blob* everyone is initially reluctant to listen to Andrews' claims, an extraterrestrial force again threatens humanity, and in a similar manner a middle-class man saves humanity.

While not strictly a Cold War film, in Steven Spielberg's *Jaws* (1975) a monster from the sea that threatens the people in town is, as with *Godzilla*, the major threat. Furthermore, one of the characters, Quint, is a shark attack survivor of the sinking of USS *Indianapolis* during World War II. Shot in Martha's Vineyard, Massachusetts, the film became a big commercial success. The motion picture is based on a novel of the same name by Peter Benchley, who also wrote the screenplay. Spielberg was initially reluctant to direct the movie but finally agreed with the condition that he would focus mainly on the shark hunt portion of the film. Footage of a real shark attack recorded by Ron and Barbara Taylor in Australia with a miniature man and a small cage (to give the illusion of a much bigger shark) was used for the movie. The role of Brody, the middle-class police officer and main protagonist, was offered to Robert Duvall but he refused, and after that Charlton Heston showed an interest in the role, but Spielberg felt Heston's persona was too grand to portray a community police officer. Finally, Roy Scheider was cast. The now classic John Williams' bass theme song earned him an Academy Award. The shots from the perspective of the shark (initially made to avoid expense) have influenced many other horror movies in the following decades.

In the film, during the hot summer of Amity Island in Massachusetts, police chief Brody discovers the remains of a shark attack victim. Initially he attempts to close the beach but the mayor is reluctant since the town's major income is based on the summer tourism activity. After a few more fatalities from shark attacks and a failed attempt to find the shark, Brody, Captain Quint and Matt Hooper, a shark expert from the Oceanographic Institute, initiate a hunt in the *Orca* for the great white. Perhaps the most terrifying scene is the moment during the hunt in which the great white shark jumps onto the boat, devouring Quint.

Politically, the film has been loosely associated with the Watergate scandal, in which a middle-class white man restores calm. The Cold War was, however, still a concern in the 1970s and a sense of paranoia is felt in the film.

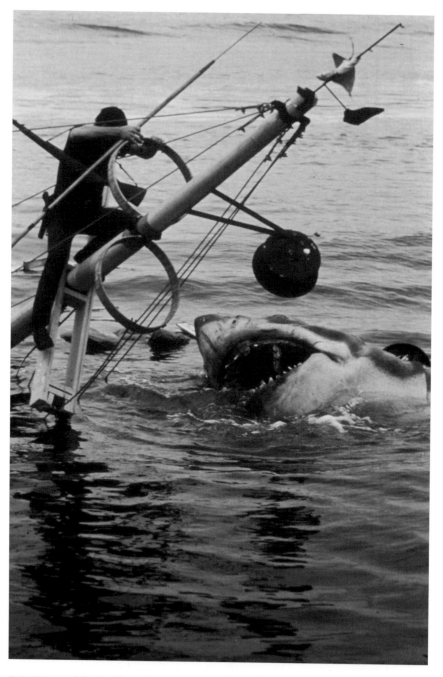

FIGURE 5.1 Middle Class Man, Chief Brody, Attempts to Save Society from a Perceived Threat (*Jaws*) © NBCUniversal

The threat may come back; in fact a few sequels were made. Mother Nature can always take revenge. *Jaws* caused mass hysteria about the uncertainty of the sea that affected several generations. For decades a fear of being attacked by a shark during the summer while swimming at the beach has remained in our collective unconscious. The fear of the water, the feeling of defenselessness and vulnerability when not in our natural medium, is a central topic of the movie. What's hiding under the sea when we are swimming? What can we encounter? A jellyfish, a puffer fish, a sea urchin, a shark? Better not to even think about it!

The *Rocky* franchise was another iconic film saga of the late 70s and 80s. In *Rocky IV* (1985), after defeating Russian boxer Ivan Drago, Rocky Balboa, draped with an American flag, gives a reconciliatory speech referencing the tension between the USA and the USSR. This film reflected the beginning of the end of the Cold War in 1985. A few months after *Rocky IV*, there was a joke in Hollywood that Rocky had run out of opponents on this planet and he would probably have to fight an alien. Based on this joke, Jim and John Thomas wrote a script about a man fighting an alien in the jungle. Arnold Schwarzenegger agreed to participate with the condition of including an entire team of special forces with him instead of just one man versus alien. For that, in order to honor the original idea that originated the film, Carl Weathers, who had played Apollo Creed in *Rocky*, was cast, among others. *Predator* (1987) is set in the jungle of Central America, a common setting of tensions during the Cold War. A special forces group of the US Army lands in a helicopter with the intention of rescuing an American official who has been kidnapped by the guerrillas. The commandos, however, run across a number of hanging bodies devoid of skin. Whoever did that does not seem to be human. Soon they discover that they are being attacked by an evil alien with four mandibles and the ability to become invisible. The alien begins killing each member of the team but a smart Schwarzenegger discovers that he can make himself invisible to the creature by hiding his body temperature, covering himself with mud.

Predator is one of the last Hollywood films to directly refer to the Cold War. Thanks to the efforts of Mikhail Gorbachev after assuming presidency of the USSR in 1985, the fall of the Berlin Wall in 1989, and the gradual and peaceful steps to independence of the countries that formed the Soviet Union in 1991, the Cold War was coming to an end.

CHAPTER 6

Witchcraft and the Worship of the Devil

WITCHCRAFT PRACTICE INVOLVES BELIEF in the use of black magic to cause an involuntary effect on a person. For centuries, witchcraft has had pejorative connotations and for the most part has been condemned by society. Across different periods, witches were accused of practicing infanticide and cannibalism and stealing penises. A witchcraft session could involve invoking Satan, who could manifest in the form of a goat. Hallucinogens from toads or other sources could be used for the rite.

During the Middle Ages hysteria about the practice of witchcraft grew among the general population. Authorities blamed witches for plagues and misfortunes. The alarm became even more prominent during the Renaissance. In 1486, Heinrich Kramer and James Sprenger published their famous book *Malleus Maleficarum* (Hammer of the Witches). Kramer worked on the book after his own failed attempt to carry a witchcraft prosecution in Innsbruck, Austria. The book was divided into three sections: Section I explored the questionable reality of witchcraft practice as a matter of fact, concluding that if the Devil is real, witchcraft must therefore be real as well. Section II explained that witches are mainly women and included a description of different witchcraft practices, and how witches can take advantage and manipulate people who may innocently seek their help. Lastly, Section III guided the reader through the legal steps needed to start a witchcraft prosecution, including interrogations, court procedures and so on.

The hysteria over witchcraft soon spread throughout all European countries and later the United States. For instance, in 1610, in Spain, Juan Valle Alvarado from the Inquisition tribunal of Logroño (La Rioja) accused up to 300 people from the Basque Country, Soria, Navarre and Burgos. Among the accused, most were women but nonetheless there were also some men, children and a priest. As a result of the trial, twelve people were executed by burning as an *auto-de-fé*, or public penance. Five of them were executed symbolically since they were already dead as a result of the torture conducted to extract their confessions. Inspired by this event, motivated young inquisitor and lawyer Alonso de Salazar Frías went to Zugarramurdi (Navarra, Spain) in search of evidence of witchcraft practice. He investigated a cave with a stream in the area said to be a witches' meeting place. He gathered almost 2,000 individuals and took testimonies while at the site. Most of the accounts were made by children and adolescents, accusing up to 5,000 people. Due to the popularity of the event, the Basque word for Sabbath, *Akelarre*, was used all over Spain to mean witchcraft practice.

Despite the attention that Inquisition trials have received, most European witch trials took place in Germany. Among the most notorious were the Trier trials (1581–1593); which resulted in an estimated 1,000 deaths; the Fulda trials (1603–1606) with around 250 deaths, and the Wurzburg trials (1626–1631) that took the lives of 157 women, children and men who were staked and burnt. Within the same period and contemporary to these trials, in the Bamberg trials (1626–1631) one of the victims was the former mayor of the town, Johannes Junius, who, after repeatedly denying the false accusations and asking for the opportunity to challenge the witnesses, was forced to confess under torture. Prior to his execution, he wrote a letter to his daughter that has been preserved. In the letter, the mayor informs his daughter that he confessed only to escape the great anguish and the bitter torture of which he had been a victim.

In the United States, the most well-known accusation of witchcraft took place in Salem, Massachusetts, between 1692 and 1693, where more than 150 colonists were accused of witchcraft. The trials resulted in nineteen people (fourteen women and five men) being hanged and one man being crushed to death. Again, many of the alleged witnesses of witchcraft practice were children and the cases were based on flimsy evidence or spectral evidence (such as dreams and visions of the spirit of the alleged witch).

In contrast to the thousands of executions due to allegations of witchcraft practice in Continental Europe during the Renaissance (especially in Germany), in the United States witchcraft accusations were rare. The famous witchcraft outbreak of Salem started innocently after two children, twelve-year-old Abigail Williams and ten-year-old Betty Parris, were playing at fortune telling about their future husbands with the then famous game the "Venus glass." The game consisted of interpreting the shapes of an egg after dropping it in a glass to predict the future, something known in history as oomancy or divinization of the egg. Soon after, the two girls began to show symptoms of agitation, flailing of their arms, and unusual postures. Betty's uncle, Reverend Parris, took the girls to physician William Griggs who did not find a medical explanation and suggested they could be victims of witchcraft practice. Parris then suggested his slave Indian woman Tituba bake a witch cake with rye and the girls' urine and feed it to a dog. If the animal showed similar signs, that would be evidence of witchcraft practice. Shortly other girls in the village, including twelve-year-old Ann Putnam Jr. and seventeen-year-old Elizabeth Hubbard, began to show similar signs of witchcraft victimization. This led to the first three accusations of witchcraft practice: against Tituba, Sarah Good and Sarah Osborne.

These three were classical victims of these types of accusations. Tituba was an Indian slave; Good was a beggar living in poverty; and Osborne had remarried an Irish man after becoming a widow, did not go to church and had legal issues with the Putnam family. While Good and Osborne denied the accusations, Tituba admitted to being the "Devil's servant." She stated that a tall man dressed all in black came to them, demanding they sign their names in a great book. She said there were other names in that book and also said that Good had ordered her cat to attack Elizabeth Hubbard, causing the scratches and bite marks on the girl's body. The young accusers agreed. By pleading guilty and collaborating, Tituba was put in jail but released after the trials ended. However, Good and Osborne, who claimed innocence, were imprisoned and sentenced to death. The act of pleading guilty while accusing others could save the indicted from execution.

As a result, up to forty people were expediently accused of witchcraft and sorcery. To deal with the increasing number of accusations, Governor Phips created a special court of oyer and terminer (hear and determine), naming William Stoughton as chief magistrate despite him having no formal legal education. Stoughton belonged to the Puritan Church. Puritans believed the English Church had been only partially reformed since the separation from the Catholic Church. Because of that opinion, they were trying to "purify" the Church from all Catholic practices. Puritans believed that Jesus Christ was above all other figures (like the Virgin Mary or the saints). They also believed in education so that anyone could read the Bible and gave special importance to the role of the family in order to facilitate devotion to God. Puritans publicly punished drunkenness and sexual relations outside of marriage. Puritanism became very popular in colonial New England. Since then, Puritan values have been deeply rooted in American values and culture. Like most Christian religions, Puritans believed in demonic forces, possessions and witchcraft. Furthermore, Stoughton was a close friend of the two influential Bostonian Puritan ministers, Increase Mather and his son Cotton Mather, author of *The Invisible Wonders of the World*.

Together with Stoughton, a number of judges were appointed to the court of oyer and terminer. While those initially accused were from lower social classes, over time respected community members were also accused and sentenced to death. Stoughton became well known for his zealous methods. When Rebecca Nurse, an elderly woman highly regarded in the community, was ruled innocent by the jury, Stoughton ordered them to reconsider their decision. After that, Nurse was declared guilty and sentenced to death. An extraordinary case was the accusation of Giles Corey who knew the law and declined to enter a plea by not stating either guilt or innocence. The judges attempted to make him plea by a process called peine forte et dure. In this process the prisoner lay naked under a table and was pressed with rocks until he made a plea. Legend has it that prior to his death two days later Corey's last words were: "More weight."

The evidence of witchcraft practice was based on the testimonies of the accusers and alleged witnesses. Stoughton and the judges decided to accept accusations based on spectral evidence, that is to say, based on the deeds committed by the spirits of the accused. While Stoughton had been advised by Increase Mather not to use spectral evidence alone, since the Devil could well trick them by taking the form of an innocent person, Stoughton believed that God would not allow the Devil to do such a thing, therefore, for him, spectral evidence was enough for building an argument of witchcraft practice. Other forms of accusation could be based on finding special ointments, remedies, books or horoscopes in the witch's possession as well as examination of the skin for lesions characteristic of what were termed "Devil's marks" or "witch's marks." It was believed that the Devil would confirm his pact with a witch by giving her or him a mark of identification. Devil's marks included a variety of skin lesions described as flat or raised, red, blue, or brown lesions, sometimes with unusual outlines.

At some point nearly half of the people in town had been accused and the court's methods were put into question. For instance, John Hathorne usually started by assuming that the accused was guilty. The situation was spiraling out of control and led to growing criticism among the locals. Finally, even the governor's wife, Lady Mary Phips, was accused. Soon afterwards, the governor forbade the use of spectral evidence and decided to dissolve the court of oyer and terminer entirely. Stoughton responded to this decision with rage, and ordered the execution of all suspected witches who were exempted by their pregnancy. Governor Phips denied enforcement of the order, causing Stoughton to leave the bench. Shortly afterwards, all the people imprisoned based on spectral evidence were released.

The circumstances leading to the Salem accusations may be explained as a case of witchcraft hysteria. In Europe there had been multiple cases over the centuries. While classically in Europe alleged witches were executed by being burnt alive at the stake, the witches of Salem were executed by hanging. This likely reflects the relative rarity of witch hunts in New England at the time. While intoxication with ergots from rye bread has been proposed as a possible explanation for the demonic visions in the accusations based on spectral evidence, this is less likely the case here with such a high number of accusations. Instead, hysteria, group paranoia or in more specific terms shared psychotic disorder seems more likely (as described in the *Diagnostic and Statistical Manual of Mental Disorders* – DSM). The young girls that began the accusations showed pseudoneurological signs and seizure-like activity. According to Dr. Griggs, these were not compatible with a medical or organic disease. As a result, based on these data, these girls most likely had some type of conversion disorder.

The Salem trials were not exempt from contemporary criticism. For instance, Judge Nathaniel Saltonstall refused to participate in the trials after being assigned by Governor Phips as one of the judges. Thomas Brattle, a Boston merchant, witnessed one of the trials and wrote a letter to an English clergyman presenting an argument against the legal premises and procedures involved in the afflictions, accusations and executions, with a particular focus on the validity of spectral evidence in proceedings. A few years after the executions, Magistrate Samuel Sewall and accuser Ann Putnam Jr. publicly apologized for their involvement in the trials. That was not the case of William Stoughton, who never apologized for his deeds.

For Stoughton, the dissolution of the court of oyer and terminer probably meant a narcissistic injury, an attack against his judgment and leadership. If proved wrong, he would have to face public shame.

Depictions and engravings of witchcraft practice were included in some of the textbooks in which witches are depicted offering children to the Devil, kissing the Devil's anus, and practicing black magic. Perhaps the most popular depictions are the ones painted by Francisco de Goya (1746–1828). In *Akelarre* (Witches' Sabbath) a group of witches gathered in a field are offering children to the Devil in the form of a goat. In *Witches' Flight*, three flying witches wearing *coroza* (penitential garments) are about to suck the blood of their victim. In Goya's series *Black Paintings*, Satan in the form of a black goat seems to be giving instructions to the witches.

Witchcraft accusations have often been seen as one of the greatest examples of mass hysteria in society. Scholars are now more inclined to believe that these accusations were used as a scapegoat to distract attention. Most of the alleged witches were victims of false accusations from their enemies, political rivals, or perhaps as on many other occasions people accused their lenders to get rid of a debt. Nevertheless, the majority of the victims of false witchcraft accusations were outcasts, marginalized people of the community, homeless, gypsies, prostitutes and the mentally ill.

Swedish film director Benjamin Christensen directed the silent film *Häxan* in 1922. He got the idea after finding a copy of the infamous *Malleus Maleficarum* in Berlin, Germany in 1919. He studied the book for nearly two years before taking the initiative for his documentary film about medieval witchcraft trials and their victims. Christensen's film became the most expensive Swedish movie of the silent era. Due to its portrayal of nudity and torture scenes the film was banned in the United States. *Häxan's* cinematography is inspired by the engravings and paintings of witchcraft during the Middle Ages in an attempt to offer a portrait of medieval culture, thought

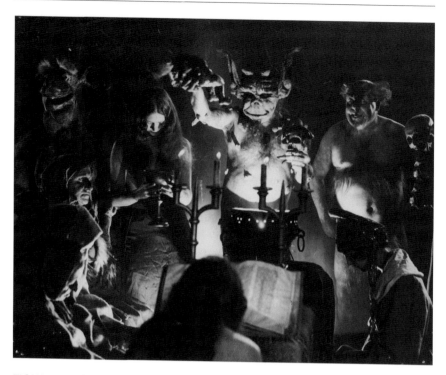

FIGURE 6.1 A Group of Witches Offering a Child to the Devil in Häxan (*Häxan*)

and attitude. The film shows pictures of witches kissing the anus of the Devil, nuns playing with Satan (played by the director), and a number of people with clear symptoms of mental illness who are being judged and sentenced to death, suggesting that most people accused of witchcraft practice in the Middle Ages were mentally ill.

In 1957, Jacques Tourneur was commissioned to direct the British film *Night of the Demon*, based on the story written by Charles Bennett. In the film, Professor Harrington attempts to expose the dangers of a Satanic sect led by Dr. Julian Karswell but is electrocuted trying to escape from a giant demonic beast that appears in the woods. After that, American psychologist Dr. John Holden arrives in the area for a conference and becomes interested in the case of Rand Hobart (a member of Karswell's sect who was accused of Harrington's murder, now in a catatonic state). Guided by Professor Harrington's notes he finds in the library of the British Museum the book *The True Discoveries of Witches and Demons*. A skeptical Holden goes to interview Karswell, and during their conversation Karswell gives him a parchment, curses him and informs him he has only three more days to live. Holden is skeptical and does not believe him but soon he begins to have misperceptions that test his emotional and mental state. In a hypnosis session they take Rand Hobart out of his catatonia with the use of stimulants. Hobart reveals that he was chosen to die from the curse but he passed it to someone else. Holden now begins to fear for his life and believes that the curse is real and realizes that he holds the parchment with the ancient inscriptions (the same as the ones in Stonehenge, and the ones that Harrington had). He starts to look for Karswell and finds him on a train trying to escape the city. Holden sneaks the parchment into his pocket, and when Karswell finds the parchment it flies from his grasp. As he chases it over the railway tracks the three-day curse expires and a giant demon arrives to slash him and toss his body on the tracks. When workers find his body it appears that he was struck by a train.

The film contains several elements of black magic, sorcery and Devil worship, in addition to the hypnotic techniques used by Dr. Holden in dealing with the catatonic patient Rand Hobart. Catatonia is a condition first described in 1874 by German psychiatrist Karl Kahlbaum (1828–1899). It was characterized by stupor, immobility and mutism. Catatonia can also present with associated symptoms such as repetition of sounds, words (echolalia) or the movements of others (echopraxia). The patients described in Oliver Sacks' memoir and later motion picture *Awakenings* (1990) suffer from catatonia secondary to encephalitis lethargica, an infectious disease of the brain. In psychiatry, catatonia has been traditionally linked to schizophrenia; in fact a subtype of this disease was called catatonic schizophrenia. However, more recent research suggests that catatonia is more frequent in mood disorders (such as unipolar or bipolar depression) rather than in primary psychotic disorders (such as schizophrenia or delusional disorders). In the film, the patient receives injections that help him come out of his catatonic state. In current psychiatric practice, an injection of lorazepam (rather than a stimulant), a type of anxiolytic medication from the family of benzodiazepines, is the gold standard treatment for catatonia.

In 1929 in Italy a new form of thriller literature was about to mark the path of a new type of horror cinema. *Giallo* (yellow) is a term that refers to a type of thriller genre in Italy based on the popular book series with a yellow cover published by Arnoldo Mondadori. The book series remained popular for decades and though some were written by Italian authors, many were translations of British or American suspense novels.

In the realms of cinema, the giallo genre was characterized by having a female protagonist who witnesses some kind of paranormal phenomena. Sexuality and eroticism were present in most films and likely due to the Catholic cultural background, the virgin was usually the sole survivor. These principles also marked Hollywood's slash killer genre. One of the first directors to bring international awareness of this kind of film genre was Mario Bava. His directorial debut in 1960, *Black Sunday* (*La Maschera del Demonio*), based on Nikolai Gogol's horror short story "Viy," became a commercial success and consolidated his directorial career.

Set in Moldavia in 1630, in *Black Sunday* Asa is sentenced to die by burning at the stake by a group of monks, after allegations of black magic practice. Prior to that a metal mask that has spikes inside is hammered into her face. Some 200 years later, a physician named Dr. Thomas Kruvajan and his assistant, Gorobec, are traveling in Moldavia for a conference and have to stop due to a problem with their car. There, they find Asa's tomb in an old crypt and remove her mask. The doctor accidentally cuts himself, dropping blood on her face, which reanimates the body (an idea also used by Clive Barker in *Hellraiser*, 1987). After that, the witch is able to find her descendants with the help of her servant whom she manipulates telepathically. One of her descendants, Katia, is exactly the age she had been before she died and has an almost identical appearance. Asa plans to drink Katia's blood to attain immortality. Prior to that, she turns the skeptical Dr. Kruvajan into a vampire. Assistant Gorobec finds out about Asa's plan and tries to stop her, but Asa attempts to make him believe she is Katia. Gorobec is able to discern between the two thanks to a crucifix Katia used to wear and this way he is able to stop the witch's plans. Finally, Asa is sentenced to die by burning at the stake one more time.

The film mixes elements of witchcraft sorcery and black magic with vampirism and eroticism. The female protagonist is obviously a seductive, very good-looking woman. She seduces and hypnotizes the doctor and turns him into a vampire with a kiss. *Black Sunday* portrays a witch-vampire who can be only killed with the traditional methods of the *Malleus Maleficarum*. Congruent with the giallo genre, the crucifix (a Catholic cult object) allows Gorobec to differentiate the witch from the virgin. The witch is resuscitated with the use of blood and immediately starts to seduce men in order to suck their blood.

In 1985, the director's son, Lamberto Bava, used elements of this film in *Demons*. In this film a girl, a prostitute, scratches herself with a display mask prior to entering the theater. The scratch turns her into a bloodthirsty demon that spreads her infection to the others watching the film.

Acclaimed director Roman Polanski directed *Repulsion* in 1965. The film tells the story of a young woman who after her sister goes on vacation is left alone in her apartment in London and gradually becomes psychotic. *Repulsion* is likely the film that best depicts the prodromal symptoms that precede a psychotic outbreak. Three years later *Rosemary's Baby* (1968) was set in the famous New York City's Dakota Building, called the Bramford in the movie. The Dakota was constructed between 1880 and 1884 in the Upper West Side of Manhattan. Architect Henry Harderbergh was inspired by the Northern German Renaissance castles. The building has hosted several celebrities, artists and musicians, including John Lennon and Yoko Ono.

The film is a story about young and beautiful Rosemary, just married to a handsome actor, Guy. The happy couple moves to a new apartment at the Bramford. Rosemary is a naïve happily married woman who is hoping to get pregnant soon. Her husband is a Broadway actor who struggles to find good roles. Soon after moving to their new apartment, Rosemary meets Terry at the laundry, a recovering drug addict who lives with an old couple, the Castevets. Terry shows her a charming amulet they gave her. That night Rosemary and Guy return home to discover that Terry has jumped out the window, apparently committing suicide. The couple meets Minnie and Roman Castevet, who don't seem very affected by their loss. That night they invite Rosemary and Guy for dinner and soon the two couples befriend each other. After dinner, Minnie gives Terry's good luck charm to Rosemary. Gradually, Rosemary begins to notice something strange about the Castevets, something that her husband does not seem to notice. As Guy begins to form a stronger bond with them, he commits to having a baby with Rosemary. Coincidentally, Guy gets the main role in the play he pursued because the producers' first choice for the character inexplicably becomes blind.

The night Guy and Rosemary plan to conceive, Minnie brings chocolate mousse and drugs Rosemary. In a dream-like state with hallucinations, Rosemary can see a group of naked people including her husband and the Castevets surrounding them. The Devil, depicted as an anthropomorphic beast with yellow eyes, comes and copulates with her. The next morning, Rosemary is still confused and talks to her husband about her experience but he calms her by telling her she passed out early in the night. Guy tells her that he had sex with her despite her being unconscious because he did not want to miss the opportunity.

Once Rosemary gets pregnant the Castevets recommend a gynecologist they trust, Dr. Abraham Sapirstein. This doctor makes her take alternative prenatal remedies, which make her crave meat and chicken liver and give her abdominal pains. When Rosemary's friend Hutch sees her in that state, he begins to do some research and discovers that she is a victim of witchcraft. Hutch unexpectedly dies but has left the book for her. Reading it, Rosemary discovers that Roman Castevet is the son of Steven Marcato (a former Satanist who lived in the building) and convinced Guy to impregnate her with Satan in exchange for guaranteeing him professional success. Desperate, she goes to her former gynecologist Dr. Hill to reveal her story, asking for help. Believing that she is delusional, Dr. Hill calls Dr. Sapirstein and her husband who take her back to the Bramford and sedate her. Rosemary delivers the baby but the next day she is told that she had a miscarriage. However, after hearing the cries of a baby from the neighbors', she grabs a knife and enters their apartment. In the first room she finds Goya's painting *Witches Sabbath*. In the next one she finds a gathering of people from different nations, the Castevets, other neighbors, and Dr. Sapirstein and her husband around a black cradle and a cross hanging upside down – an allegory of the Antichrist. Rosemary is initially horrified to see that the creature has yellow eyes. However, Roman Castevet encourages her to be a mother for him. Rosemary is initially hesitant but finally agrees.

The film represents the converse of the advent of Christ. With the help of witches, Satan chooses a mortal woman to conceive a son in this world: the Antichrist. The film portrays psychiatric symptoms that can occur during pregnancy. Anxiety, including worrying excessively, panic symptoms with palpitations, muscle tension, dizziness, shortness of breath, gastrointestinal symptoms, or intrusive thoughts are fairly common. Also mood symptoms, sadness, and dysphoria can occur. Psychotic symptoms such as delusional beliefs or persecution paranoia, suspicion of poisoning, and hallucinations can be seen as well in extreme cases. Women with a history of psychiatric disorders in prior pregnancies are at especial risk, but the symptoms may occur in individuals with no history of mental ill health. The onset of psychiatric symptoms can be postpartum as well. In this case, *Rosemary's Baby* can be seen as the portrayal of a woman with possibly normal premorbid anxiety who starts to become gradually more anxious and dysphoric during her pregnancy, escalating to a psychotic episode with delusional symptoms of persecution and poisoning. Despite the film suggesting her experiences are in fact real, from a psychiatric viewpoint Rosemary displays anxiety, mood and psychotic symptoms that may occur during pregnancy.

Historically, witchcraft practice was related to the use of hallucinogenic substances. The chocolate mousse of the Castevets given prior to the copulation ritual with the Devil could well have contained a hallucinogen. Psychedelic drugs were popular in the 60s and, just as when Rosemary copulates with the Devil, they can alter the perception of senses, space and time.

Before making *Superman* (1978), Richard Donner started his career directing horror film *The Omen* (1976). It stars Gregory Peck as Robert (an American diplomat living in Rome) who after finding that his wife, Katherine, has had a stillbirth, agrees to a priest's offer and adopts the child of a mother who had died during delivery at the same time. Nevertheless, Robert keeps this a secret from his wife. Their child is named Damien. Soon Robert is appointed US Ambassador to Great Britain and the family moves to London. Early in his development, Damien's behavior diverges from what is normally expected in addition to other abnormal qualities. Animals seem scared of him and he is for some reason extremely resistant to entering a church. Damien seems to have some kind of supernatural talent for telekinesis and hypnotizing people into behaving according to his will. On his fifth birthday, his nanny hangs herself for him in front of all the assistants. Later, a strange nanny called Mrs. Baylock, who claims to have come from the agency, shows up at the house to become Damien's caretaker. A Catholic priest tells Robert that Damien is not human and that his wife is pregnant and Damien won't allow the birth of the new child. The priest is later killed by a lightning rod thrown from the roof of a church. Keith, a photographer who had taken pictures of the nanny, and the father realize that the victims have some strange pointing shadows in the photos that somehow presage their fatal destiny.

In the meantime, Damien rides his tricycle at home and pushes his mother downstairs, causing her miscarriage. At the hospital, Katherine, not knowing anything about Damien's origins, tells Robert that she is scared of her son.

Robert and Keith travel to Rome to investigate Damien's origins and find that the hospital he was born in has been destroyed by fire. The agonizing father who offered Robert the child writes the name of an Etruscan cemetery where the body of Damien's mother lies. Keith and Robert go to the cemetery, exhume the body and discover that Damien's mother was a jackal. Next to the jackal they find Robert's biological son who was killed at birth so that he could take Damien. After that they realize Damien is the Antichrist coming to the world to start an evil empire with the help of a group of Satanists. After escaping the attack of a group of Rottweilers they leave the cemetery and fly to Israel to meet with Carl Bugenhagen, an expert on the Antichrist who advises them to kill Damien in a ritualistic manner. Robert is hesitant but Keith sees no other solution; however, he is killed by falling glass. In the meantime, Mrs. Baylock goes to visit Katherine at the hospital and throws her out of the window.

After returning to London, frustrated with the murders, Robert kills Mrs. Baylock and takes Damien to a church to kill him. However, he has been followed by a police officer due to his reckless driving who is able to shoot him before he stabs Damien. The boy is later seen at his father's funeral holding the hand of the US president.

Damien's behavior is consistent with conduct disorder, a psychiatric condition characterized by a behavioral pattern of aggression towards others, breaking of rules, vandalism and truancy. This disorder usually starts early in childhood and is required for a later diagnosis of antisocial personality disorder – the so-called psychopaths – in later adulthood. As in the case of Damien, children with conduct disorder seem to have a lack of empathy for others' suffering. Damien does not hesitate to kill his own nanny and mother to achieve his goals. He is vehemently opposed to entering the church. Though conduct disorder has been related to neglect and abuse, recent evidence suggests a strong component of inheritance. Children with conduct disorder tend to have a lack of reward pleasure in the orbitofrontal cortex (the area of the brain just above the orbit), a low basal heart rate related to new sensation, and hyposensitivity to pleasure. As in *The Omen*, even if adopted by good nurturing parents, children of people with antisocial personality tend to develop similar behavioral patterns, even when psychosocial risk factors have been removed from their environment. As he grows, Damien will go on to kill whoever is a potential obstacle in his path to power. He shows no remorse.

Similarly to *The Omen*, Lynne Ramsay's film *We Need to Talk about Kevin* (2011) narrates the story of a child with conduct disorder who, despite having all the psychosocial elements for a good healthy development, kills his entire family and commits a massacre at his school with a bow and arrows.

In both *The Omen* and *We Need to Talk about Kevin*, we can see how their mothers notice something strange with their children, as if they lacked the human quality of empathy, and are perhaps the reincarnation of the Devil.

Together with Mario Bava, Dario Argento was one of the major directors of giallo cinema. Argento's masterpiece *Suspiria* (1977) was praised by many critics due to its cinematography. For *Suspiria*, Argento found inspiration in the German Expressionist movement and in Walt Disney's cartoon film *Snow White and the Seven Dwarfs* (1937), a film that he had seen as a child and had found very scary. To honor the Disney movie, Argento filmed using Technicolor, a technique developed by Walt Disney for *Snow White*. The use of color and flashes in the film lead the viewer through an almost hallucinatory experience. From a psychodynamic perspective, perhaps Argento became eroticized by the fear experienced while watching *Snow White*, something that led him to become one of the greatest horror film directors of all time.

In *Suspiria*, Suzy Bannion is an American ballet dancer who travels to Germany to study at a prestigious dance academy in Freiburg. There she meets Pat who is stabbed and hanged that same night by a mysterious person with a monstrous arm. Next a series of mysterious murders begin to take place at the academy. Later Suzy learns from another student that Pat died because she had discovered a secret about the institution. Finally, Suzy discovers that the academy is directed by a group of witches.

As in other giallo films, we see a young woman who suspects there is something wrong and solves the riddle of the gory murders on her own.

Based on the novel by Stephen King with the same title, *Thinner* (1996) was directed by Tom Holland. It narrates the story of overweight and ambitious lawyer Billy Halleck who uses Machiavellian methods to defend wealthy mobsters and criminals. One night driving back home after the celebration of a successful defense, he asks his wife to give him oral sex and, distracted, he accidentally runs over a gypsy woman who dies due to the inflicted injuries. Billy omits to mention in court the reason he got distracted and is found not guilty. However, the father of the gypsy woman, Tadzu Lempke, curses and put a hex on Billy in revenge, by saying the word "thinner." After that, Billy begins to unintentionally lose weight. No matter how hard he tries to eat, he continues to lose weight and become weaker. Finally, Billy is able to convince Tadzu to help him. Tadzu says that he fears for his people and only agrees to help him by giving him the possibility to transfer the curse to someone else. He puts his blood into a strawberry pie and tells him that he can get free of the hex if he is able to make an unsuspecting person eat the pie who will consequently suffer a rapid painful death. After finding out his wife was having an affair with his physician, Dr. Mike, Billy offers his wife a piece of his favorite pie. Nevertheless, the next morning he finds out that his daughter had visited from college and ate from the pie as well. In despair, Billy is about to eat a piece of the pie himself to commit suicide but is surprised by the visit of Dr. Mike. Billy then changes his mind and closes the door with a macabre smile.

The character of Billy suffers from some kind of pathological gluttony. Though obesity has been traditionally seen as a medical problem in the field of endocrinology, a psychiatric approach to understand obesity has gradually become stronger over the last decade. In that case, obesity can be classified under addictive disorders, with food being the addictive substance in this case. Recent research findings at the National Institute of Mental Health prove that neuroscientifically food can stimulate the reward system of our brain by enhancing dopamine in a similar pattern to other drugs. Moreover, obese people with food addiction go through similar episodes of bingeing, losing control, dysphoria, guilt, and continuation of the behavior despite acknowledgment of the negative consequences of it.

For many people, eating can also be a behavioral response to stress. Under acute stress, our body releases cortisol and orexins, increasing appetite and stimulating us to eat. From an evolutionary perspective, eating under stress helps us increase the reserves of our body to confront potential food scarcity. This may have been an adaptive survival strategy in the past but, nowadays, overeating under stress or anxiety can certainly be maladaptive, causing obesity and increasing the risk of diabetes, cardiovascular diseases and cancer.

Therefore, food can be as addictive as any other drug. Therapies traditionally used for the treatment of substance use disorders such as motivational interviewing, the twelve-step groups and so on can also be used for people who suffer a similar problem with food.

Sociologically, diet changes, the aggressive marketing campaigns for fast food, and the lack of availability of healthy food, together with the increase in sedentary lifestyles, have dramatically increased the incidence of obesity in children and adults. Nevertheless, society has responded by encouraging healthier lifestyles and diet choices. For instance, in psychiatry there is now a strong emphasis in the literature for the use of nutrients rich in Omega-3, polyunsaturated fatty acids, antioxidants, and unrefined carbohydrates which combined with exercise can certainly be helpful in the prevention of mental illness, its prognosis and its relapse risk.

From the view of personality disorders, *Thinner's* main character, Billy, seems to have a behavioral pattern of disregard for right and wrong, persistent lying and manipulation of others. He is egocentric and lacks empathy for others, traits of antisocial personality disorder, something that would hinder his treatment if he sought help from a physician for his weight problem.

Inspired by the Swedish movie *Häxan*, Haxan Films, a company based in Orlando, Florida produced a found footage witch film, *The Blair Witch Project* (1999). The film was directed by Eduardo Sánchez and Daniel Myrick. After Ruggero Deodato's *Cannibal Holocaust* (1980), this became the first popular found footage film and was followed by the now classic horror films *REC* (2007) and *Paranormal Activity* (2009). With the found footage filmmaking technique, one of the actors becomes the cameraperson, allowing the viewer to see through his or her eyes. This method allows more improvisation, giving a further sense of realism, adding more drama and increasing the horror and suspense.

In *The Blair Witch Project*, three students, Heather Donahue, Michael Williams and Joshua Leonard, go to the northern forest of Burkittsville, Maryland, formerly known as Blair, Maryland, to make a documentary about the Blair Witch, a woman who after being accused of witchcraft was hanged in the eighteenth century in the area. Once in town, the students hear from locals that the spirit of the witch is still around and the forest is haunted. Legend has it that a father pleaded not guilty by reason of insanity, claiming that he had been possessed by the Blair Witch after killing his children in an abandoned house in the forest. After three days in the forest, the protagonists realize they are unable to return to their car. The first few nights they hear crackling and noises but think they are made by wild animals. The panic begins to build when they see anthropomorphic stick figures hanging from the trees – an allegory of the witch executions – and hear the voices of children in the middle of the night. At some point they realize that no matter which direction they take, they always return to the same original point. One night, Josh runs away and disappears in the forest. Later, a bundle of sticks held together with pieces of his bloody shirt appears next to the other two tents. Heather finds some nails, teeth and hair but does not tell Michael. That night, following the screams of someone who appears to be Josh, they arrive at an abandoned house with handprints made by children on the walls. Following the screams that seem to come from all over the house, Heather records the body of Michael standing still but she falls before knowing what happened.

The found footage film style permits the audience to better identify with the characters' feelings and emotions, which in this case enhances the fearful feelings. From a psychological perspective, *The Blair Witch Project* can be viewed through the learned helplessness model of depression. This model was proposed by famous psychologist Martin Seligman and states that after multiple failed attempts to achieve a goal (trying to get back to the car) a person begins to think that no matter how hard they try they will fail. This cognitive model has been used to explain why people stop their attempts to pursue academic, professional or romantic success, feeling that no matter what they do they will still fail. The model was used to provide an explanation for depression and helped the development of animal models of depression. In these animal models, a mouse is put into a water pool where there is no escape. After multiple attempts to leave the pool the mouse stops trying even when it is later offered an escape route. If treated with antidepressants there will be a higher chance that they attempt to escape the pool. In the film, after multiple attempts to escape the forest going south or west the protagonists feel that no matter what they do they always arrive back at the same point. In despair they lose the motivation to keep walking. On the last night Heather makes some footage apologizing to the co-producers and their families for making the film, maybe feeling that this apology might somehow save them. In desperate situations magical or religious pleas are a very common call for help.

Director Sam Raimi and his brother, emergency physician Ivan Raimi, wrote the horror masterpiece that combines elements of witchcraft, sorcery, Satanism, possession and spiritism. *Drag Me to Hell* was finally released in 2009.

In the horror movie, Christine works as a loan manager in a local bank. Christine had grown up an obese kid in a rural area, her father died and her mother was an alcoholic. In contrast she is now a resilient, attractive, good-hearted, smart young woman who dates Clay, a young good-looking physician. At work she has a good chance of getting a promotion as an assistant manager. However, a new competitor, Stu Rubin, is willing to do anything to win the promotion too. One day, Sylvia Ganush, a one-eyed, sick-looking old gypsy woman with a phlegmatic cough, who repeatedly takes out and puts in her rotten false teeth to taste the different candies at Christine's desk, comes to ask for a third extension of her mortgage. Christine is initially willing to help this woman but feeling that this may affect her chances of getting the promotion she denies the extension. The gypsy woman does not give up and begs on her knees. After Christine calls security, the gypsy woman attacks her while blaming Christine for shaming her. The gypsy woman later waits for Christine in her car that night to attack her again. During the altercation the gypsy woman steals one of her buttons to curse her. Subsequently Christine begins to have abnormal perceptions, nightmares about the woman, anxiety, and hypervigilance. After dinner with her boyfriend she goes to visit an Indian psychic reader who tells her she has been cursed and the Lamia, a demon, will torment her for three days prior to dragging her to hell. Christine begins to panic and her boyfriend takes her to a doctor who diagnoses her with PTSD, a psychiatric disorder that involves prominent anxiety symptoms following a traumatic experience, related to the attack by the gypsy woman. This seems likely as Christine seems to be having intrusive recurrent thoughts, and symptoms of hyperarousal and hypervigilance. Nevertheless, Christine continues to experience terrifying appearances of the Lamia demon in the form of a goat. Advised by the guru she sacrifices her kitten against her principles but this does not help much. The psychic reader finally recommends a medium that can help her but for that she needs to receive $10,000. Her boyfriend does not understand anything but seeing how important it is to her, he helps her with the money. They go to see the medium Shaun San Dena, who prepares a séance. They bring a goat and plan to transfer the Lamia to the animal to kill him. However, when San Dena's assistant, Milos, is about to kill the animal, the now possessed goat bites him and the demon transfers to the assistant. Chaos erupts in the room but San Dena is able to send the spirit away. The psychic reader, however, advises Christine that the Lamia will come back and if she gives the accursed button to someone else she will be able to get rid of the problem. Christine is not willing to do that to another person but realizes she can give it to the now dead gypsy woman, thinking that the soul never dies. She goes to the cemetery and despite significant resistance from the "dead body" she is able to put it in the body's mouth. Feeling that she is now free of the curse, the next day she goes to the train station to start a deserved vacation with her boyfriend who is about to ask for her hand in marriage. However, as the train is approaching, her boyfriend brings her the button in an envelope, making her realize she mixed up her envelope with another. In shock she falls off the train platform and the Lamia opens a hole in the ground, dragging her to hell. The train is approaching and the helpless Clay can only watch with horror.

The trauma symptoms that Christine goes through after the first outbreak – recurrent intrusive thoughts during the day and in the form of nightmares at night, avoidance of reminders, increased anxiety, arousal and hypervigilance with anything that would remind her of the situation – are typical symptoms of PTSD. However, in the realms of psychiatry, for this kind of diagnosis, at least four weeks' duration of symptoms are needed. For patients who are experiencing symptoms when the trauma happened less than four weeks earlier, a diagnosis of acute stress disorder is preferred. Fortunately, most people who go through traumatic experiences don't develop PTSD. At first thought, Christine could be at higher risk because of growing up without a father and with an alcoholic mother; there is a high likelihood that she suffered neglect or abuse, and her childhood puts her in a more vulnerable position and at higher likelihood of becoming dysfunctional with new traumas. On second thought, though, Christine seems to be fully aware of her past; she does not seem to be ashamed of it. In this case, Christine seems to be a resilient person with mature defenses and good feelings. Among other causes, trauma has been proposed as a possible reason for people believing they have been possessed by a different entity. At times, overcoming difficulties becomes the key to learning and success in life. Christine seems to be doing fairly well but out of her rivalry and ambition to win the assistant manager position she will make one mistake that will destroy everything she has built.

Night of the Demon (1957) was likely a big influence on Sam Raimi's film. In both films a person is cursed and stalked for three days prior to being fatally attacked by a demon. In the two, a séance and a medium are used in an attempt to clarify or solve the problem.

Rob Zombie, the lead singer of the band White Zombie, began his career as film director with the successful *House of 1000 Corpses* (2003). His more recent project *The Lords of Salem* (2012) stars Zombie's wife, Sheri Moon

Zombie as Heidi. She is a recovering drug addict in Salem, Massachusetts who works on a local metal radio show. Heidi is the descendant of Reverend Hawthorne, a man who executed a number of witches two centuries previously. However, just before dying, one of the witches cursed the descendants of Hawthorne. Heidi's neighbors are three witches who were descendants of the original witches. One day she interviews Francis Matthias at her radio show, a man who has just written a book about the Salem witch trials. Heidi plays an album she has received anonymously at home – the music of the Lords of Salem. Francis, in his research, discovers that the music was in the documents of the Salem trials and tries to warn Heidi but he is killed by Heidi's neighbors. Then the witches play the music at the radio station to attract all the descendants of the witches in town who gather in a local theater. The next day the radio reports a mass suicide at a rock concert, and Heidi has disappeared.

Zombie's film seems aesthetically influenced by Stanley Kubrick. *The Lords of Salem* incorporates elements of sexuality with witchcraft. Mozart's "Requiem" in the background helps provide the atmosphere. Historically, witchcraft practice has been related to obscenity and unacceptable sexual behavior. In one scene, Heidi falls asleep in a church and dreams that a priest is trying to rape her. In the final scene, all the witches strip and gather at the theater. On top, there is Heidi giving birth to a creature – the Antichrist? Also set in the bewitched city of Salem, the TV show *American Horror Story: Coven* tells the story of a group of Salem witches who fled from New Orleans to escape execution.

According to folkloric tales of witchcraft practice, the Devil could take the form of a man in black or a goat. Robert Eggers collects all the traditional stories about witches in his directorial debut film *The Witch* (2015). The story is set in rural New England during the 17th century and narrates the recruitment process of a new witch. First under the form of a goat and then as a man in black, the Devil manipulates and destroys a Puritan family with the help of a witch. The Devil adopts an anthropomorphic form in *Devil* by John Dowdle (2010), based on the story by M. Night Shyamalan. In an ancient story, the Devil at times comes to Earth in human form to confine a group of sinners in a trap, taking the lives of each of them, one at a time. The story is told in a voice-over by Ramirez, one of the characters, who states that the Devil would first appear after a suicide. At that moment the voice is interrupted by a violent suicide in which a man falls onto a truck from one of the skyscrapers of Philadelphia.

Detective Bowden, who is recovering from alcohol dependence related to the loss of his wife and son, is investigating the death of this person and discovers that the man's jump onto the truck caused the truck to roll and end up a few blocks away from the scene. He finds out that in the building that the man jumped off, five other people are trapped in the elevator. These people begin to die violently every time the power of the elevator goes off. All of them have one thing in common: they all are sinners. Of all of them, the Devil turns out to be the older woman, who appears the most innocent. She is the last one in the elevator with Tony, who confesses his sin that he committed a hit and run five years earlier while driving, killing the mother and son of Detective Bowden. After the confession and his display of true remorse, the Devil is not able to take his life. Detective Bowden, however, is still able to forgive.

The content of the story has a strong Catholic flavor. To begin with, Ramirez, the person who tells the story, has a Hispanic name. This implies that his grandma's story probably originated in Mexico, Salvador, Puerto Rico or some other Hispanic country with Catholic traditions. In *Devil*, Tony – a classic Italian American name – confesses his sin and is forgiven. In Catholicism, confession is the ritual that leads towards forgiveness. No matter how bad the sin is, in Catholicism, a person can always be forgiven if, as in the film, he or she is able to show true repentance. Psychologically, the confession is an act of catharsis that relieves the sinner from the feeling of guilt.

According to the Catholic tradition, Satan was an angel who rebelled against God. In the Book of Revelation, Saint John states that Satan was cast out of heaven by God in great anger against those who disobey His commands. The Devil was also thought to take the form of the serpent that tempted Eve to eat from the apple of wisdom in the Garden of Eden. In the Middle Ages and the Renaissance multiple depictions were made of the Devil and demons as monstrous and gruesome figures in representations of hell or the temptations of the saints. Yet, during the late Renaissance, Baroque and Neoclassical periods, more images of the Devil in human form begin to appear. For example, the representation of Saint Michael and the Devil from Bartolomé Bermejo in Spain from 1468 shows the Devil as a big black demon and, in contrast, another version of the same theme by Raphael in 1505 represents the Devil as an ugly human with wings. Nonetheless, in Spain for example, this representation of the Devil coexisted with other iconographies such as the Devil as the goat portrayed in Goya's *Witches' Sabbath*.

Stories of witchcraft and the worship of the Devil became popular in Europe and spread to the United States from England. In times of moral panic, witch hunts served the purpose to restore order in society. Witch hunts generally affected people of lower socioeconomic status who lacked the resources to defend themselves. The term "witch hunt" has been used up to today to describe any mass hysteric persecution of a certain group that usually results in the harming of innocent people. That was the case with McCarthy's communist witch hunt in Hollywood and arguably the current persecution of sexual offenders in the United States.

CHAPTER 7

Demonic Possessions

A DEMONIC POSSESSION IMPLIES the invasion of a person by a demon or a supernatural force. The word "demon" comes from the Greek *daimon*. In ancient Greece, the *daimon* could be good or evil depending on their deeds, but avenging spirits were considered evil forces. The Judeo-Christian demon is the result of an integration of the Greek *daimon* with avenging spirits. In the Old Testament, the first book of Samuel tells the story of David playing the harp for Saul to alleviate the torments caused by a demon; the spirit would leave at the sound of the harp and Saul's pain would be relieved. The book of Tobit (Tobias) tells the story of Sarah, who was harassed by the demon Asmodeus who had killed seven of her husbands. Tobias was able to make the demon flee to Egypt. In the New Testament, there are many references to demonic possession and eight cases of exorcism. Among them, the story of the Gerasene demoniac stands out as one of the most detailed descriptions of demonic possession. According to the Gospels, this demoniac was living in the tombs and had been chained by hands and feet. Soon before Jesus' arrival in the city, he had broken his chains and no one was able to bide him or subdue him any more. Furthermore, he would cry out and cut himself with stones night and day. When Jesus encountered him he ordered the demon to come out of him; after the exorcism, his judgment was restored.

With the popularity of Christianity in the Roman Empire, demonic possession became an explanation for erratic behavior in society. Religious men during the Middle Ages practiced exorcisms as a way to imitate Jesus. For instance Saint Francis of Assisi performed an exorcism for a man who had convulsions and foaming from the mouth – a symptom of epilepsy.

During the early modern period, the criteria for demonic possession become more complex and restrictive. A demoniac now had to be able to speak in tongues, levitate, have unusual strength, and be able to decrease the temperature in the room where he or she was. A simple case of agitation, or seizures, would not be enough to justify a demonic possession. As a result, demonic possession syndrome becomes more likely in neurotic individuals (people with symptoms of anxiety, dissociative identity, somatoform, and personality disorders rather than with severe mental illness or epilepsy). A famous case in 1566 was that of Nicole Obry, a newly married Catholic sixteen-year-old French girl, who claimed to have seen the spirit of her grandfather while visiting his tomb at the cemetery. The spirit had told her that he was suffering in purgatory because he did not have time to confess when he died. He also said that the family had to make several pilgrimages to nearby shrines and to Santiago de Compostela so that he could be relieved from purgatory. The family made the pilgrimages to the closer shrines but not to Santiago, which resulted in Nicole suffering seizures. Furthermore, the spirit warned that if they didn't visit the tomb of the apostle, her grandfather's spirit would turn deaf, dumb and blind. At this time Nicole suffered a temporary paralysis, which made the village priest and a local teacher suspect that she had not been possessed by the grandfather's spirit but by an evil spirit. It was determined to perform a public exorcism in the cathedral of Laon. The demon Beelzebub talked trough Nicole's mouth; he claimed that the Protestant Huguenots were his friends and that together they would harm Christ even more than Jews had done. Nicole replied to questions in several foreign languages and could not resist the presence of the Eucharist due to the recognition of the real presence of Christ. To be able to get rid of the malevolent invasion, she was fed with several hosts until the demons came out of her body. This public exorcism was an attack against the Protestant Huguenots who questioned the dogma of transubstantiation. Many Huguenots returned to Catholicism, whereas others realized that the whole performance was a trick by the Catholic Church to confirm the dogma and attack its rivals.

In a short period of time, Nicole Obry suffered pseudovisual hallucinations, conversional seizures and paralysis. In this case, demonic possession could be seen as a dissociative trance disorder, and exorcism was a curative abreaction for the demoniac. This exorcism of Nicole Obry became well known and was used to support Catholicism in France over the new Protestant religions. Some form of histrionic personality disorder in Nicole and the efforts of the priest to use this opportunity could explain the theatricality of the case.

Today Catholicism and other Christian religions, such as the Pentecostals, accept demonic possession. In fact, some religious psychiatrists also accept the possibility of demonic possession as a different entity. M. Scott Peck, for example, the writer of *The Road Less Traveled*, had a close relationship with famous Irish Catholic exorcist Father Malachi Martin. Peck converted to Catholicism and with the help of a priest, practiced exorcisms for some of his patients whom he believed were demonically possessed in addition to having other psychiatric afflictions. Based on these experiences he wrote *Glimpses of the Devil: A Psychiatrist's Personal Accounts of Possession, Exorcism, and Redemption*. In this book, he writes about his personal experiences diagnosing some of his patients with demonic possession and how exorcism was beneficial. These patients also had a history of psychiatric disorders (like borderline personality disorder and schizophrenia) underlying an alleged demonic possession. For Peck, demonic possession and mental illness could happen concomitantly. In those cases, an exorcism could be beneficial in addition to the regular psychiatric treatment he provided.

Psychiatrists often encounter patients who come seeking spiritual advice for religious problems regarding their faith. However, the American Psychiatric Association states that psychiatrists should refrain from treating spiritual conflicts. Instead patients should be referred to chaplains or other spiritual advisers.

William Friedkin's *The Exorcist* (1973) starts with some excavations in Northern Iraq, one of the regions where human civilization first flourished. Father Merrin discovers a figure of the Assyrian demon Pazuzu, the king of demons of the wind. In the meantime Regan, an innocent girl in her early teens, lives in Georgetown with her mother Chris, a famous actress. Regan's parents are separated and there is still a lot of conflict between them, something Regan seems to resent. After moving to a new house, she begins to play with a Ouija board she finds in the basement and starts talking to her mother about her new friend Captain Howdy. Soon Regan begins to develop behavioral changes, urinating on the carpet in front of guests and telling them they all are going to die. Concerned, Chris takes Regan to a neurologist who prescribes Ritalin (methylphenidate) for her nerve problem, something that does not help much. Regan's bed shakes at night and what looks like a strong supernatural force swings her violently. She also develops personality changes. She begins to swear and makes obscene gestures. The neurologists believe that Regan has temporal lobe epilepsy, something that would explain her convulsions, behavior changes and hallucinations, but the electroencephalogram does not show any seizure activity. After doing a cerebral arteriogram, a pneumogram and other tests they can't find any organic cause for her syndrome. The neurologist recommends that Regan sees a psychiatrist after witnessing an episode of violent movements and seeing that Thorazine (chlorpromazine) does not make any difference. In the session, the psychiatrist hypnotizes Regan, bringing out the demon that has taken possession. At that moment, Regan grabs the psychiatrist's genitals aggressively. After this episode, she is evaluated by a group of psychiatrists who believe Regan has a delusional disorder, a kind of psychotic disorder that makes her believe she is possessed by a demon. The psychiatrists recommend inpatient admission with careful observation for weeks to months but Chris, losing patience, objects to that, so one of the psychiatrists suggests she takes her daughter to an exorcist.

One night, Chris goes out and leaves her daughter in the house under the care of her friend Burke. When Chris comes back home, she finds Regan sleeping. Her room is unusually cold. Outside, Burke is found dead a few

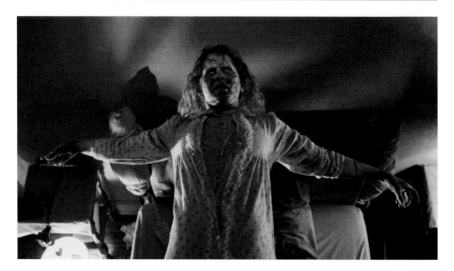

FIGURE 7.1 Young Regan Levitates Under the Possession by Demon Pazuzu
(*The Exorcist*) Licensed by Warner Bros. Entertainment Inc. All
rights reserved.

steps away from Chris's house. Detective Kinderman is assigned to investigate the murder and goes to the house to ask questions. After the detective leaves the house, Regan starts swearing; turns her head completely backwards; and, speaking with Burke's voice, reveals that she killed her friend. In despair, Chris takes steps to contact Father Karras, who is also a board-certified psychiatrist.

Father Karras's mother has Alzheimer's disease and dies after hospitalization in a psychiatric institution with poor resources. Father Karras's brother blames him for not having pursued his career as a psychiatrist, something that could have made him more wealthy and successful. After his mother's death, Father Karras is in the midst of a crisis of faith, something he shares with another priest while they smoke a cigarette and drink a glass of bourbon.

When Chris approaches Father Karras, he is initially reluctant to believe that Regan is demonically possessed, and tells Chris that exorcisms are obsolete and no one practices them any more. For Father Karras demonic possessions are a manifestation of mental illnesses such as schizophrenia or conversive reactions. However, after meeting with Regan and hearing a recording backwards in which Regan is asking for help, he agrees to perform an exorcism with the help of Father Merrin, an experienced exorcist.

When Father Merrin and Father Karras start to recite the ritual of exorcism, Regan manifests several abnormal phenomena: she is able to move objects using telekinesis, speak ancient languages, and levitate. She has unusual strength, an abnormally long tongue and projectile vomits. At some point, Regan talks to Father Karras in the voice of his mother, which makes him break down, but Father Merrin sends him away. When Father Karras returns, he finds Father Merrin dead on the floor. Furiously, he grabs the young girl and shouts at the demon, commanding him to take him instead. The demon Pazuzu obeys and, after discovering that he has been possessed by the evil spirit, Father Karras immediately commits suicide by hurling himself through the window.

The Exorcist was based on the novel of the same name by William Peter Blatty. The novel was inspired by the true story of Roland Doe, a fourteen-year-old boy who was believed to be possessed by the Devil in 1949. While hospitalized in the psychiatric wing of Georgetown University Hospital, the boy rejected several sacred objects, made objects fly and his bed shake. Three Catholic priests performed up to thirty exorcisms over several weeks. After the exorcisms, the boy did not remember anything, grew up healthy, got married and had children and grandchildren. The film instead is narrated in the 1970s (at that time, the present) and though it was made consistent with the original story (it was set in Georgetown, Washington DC), a young girl was chosen as the subject of demonic possession, adding more drama.

Possession syndrome is characterized by a supernatural force taking control over the human body. This phenomenon has been described across all continents throughout history. Perhaps the most common disease associated with exorcism was epilepsy. As depicted in Friedkin's film, Regan manifests tonic-clonic convulsions, and her eyes roll back, something typical in grand mal seizures. Behavioral and personality changes, hyperreligiosity or obscenity, and delusions or hallucinations have been more consistently described in temporal lobe seizures (as suggested by the neurologist). Non-goal-directed violence is more common in partial complex seizures. In the absence of a primary neurological disorder, the symptoms shown by Regan could be explained in the context of mania (an episode of bipolar disorder). Increased agitation, hyperactivity, decreased sleep and increased strength are symptoms of this condition. Regan also shows symptoms of psychosis involving delusions and hallucinations (something compatible with bipolar mania as well). Another possible diagnosis is Tourette's disorder, a type of tic disorder in which coprolalia, a compulsion to swear, is a possibility. As explained earlier, during the Early Modern period, the criteria required for demonic possession became more complex and specific: speaking in tongues, making unnatural body postures, creating a cold feeling in the room, and rejecting religious images. Regan manifests all these symptoms. Since genuine demonic possession is not a conceivable diagnosis in the field of psychiatry, some compatible psychiatric diagnoses here would be dissociative identity (a neurosis in which a person has two identities, the good Regan and the evil demonically possessed Regan) and/or conversion disorder (a disturbance characterized by neurological symptoms – seizures – without physical findings). Personality wise, histrionic personality disorder (a pattern of emotional excessiveness and attention-seeking behaviors) is the most common.

In some cases of demonic possessions of a neurotic nature, exorcism could be therapeutic as an abreaction, a type of catharsis. An exorcism could help induce a trance state and an enhancement of consciousness that could potentially be curative. In that case, if Regan's beliefs are of a neurotic rather than a psychotic nature, she could potentially be cured by performing an exorcism. Neurotic disorders such as conversion disorder, dissociative disorder and anxiety disorders are characterized by distress without loss of function and preservation of contact with reality. In those scenarios, hypnosis or psychoanalytic therapies have been helpful historically. In fact some scholars believe that hypnotherapy was developed from the exorcism techniques proposed by Father Gassner in the eighteenth century. In Regan's case, an exorcism could help the release of an unconscious inner conflict (such as distress related to her parents' separation or some kind of traumatic sexual memory) and cathartically heal her symptoms.

In addition to Regan's circumstances, there are other aspects of *The Exorcist* that are interesting for psychiatric discussion. Father Karras abandoned psychiatry to become a priest but after losing his mother he is having a crisis of faith. After significant stressful situations a change in our belief system can happen. Often people have a religious response to stress, praying more, or pleading for help to a higher power. In extreme cases, some people can have a hyperreligious awakening, as with the so-called born again Christians. In other cases it can go the other way around, involving a loss of faith, and a turn to agnosticism or atheism and logical thinking (as in the case of Father Karras). In contrast to Father Karras's crisis, Chris does not seem much interested in faith or religion; she just wants to help her daughter. Chris is a famous person, and has multiple resources that allow her to go to prestigious professionals. However, sometimes famous people receive poorer treatment than average. In these situations, described in the literature as the VIP syndrome, due to fame, money, power or position, care is disrupted by the special treatment the person receives from the team. When such clinical scenarios occur, the regular care of a patient gradually shifts away from the expected medical care towards a new friendly relationship. This increases the risk of neglecting medical routine care in benefit of the new friendly interaction. This is usually due to the physician's inner motivations to be liked by the VIP person and the way the VIP usually interacts with people in the world. However, despite the fact Regan is a VIP patient (the daughter of a famous actress) there is no evidence of VIP syndrome in the interaction with the doctors. Nevertheless, Chris seems to be used to getting whatever she wants and when frustrated shows maladaptive defenses, which don't facilitate the doctors' work.

A few years after the success of *The Exorcist*, the low budget independent film about possessions, *The Evil Dead* (1981), was released and soon gained a cult following. The film was directed by Sam Raimi and starred Bruce

Campbell. Both had become friends during the 70s and had envisioned working on a film together. *The Evil Dead* (1981) tells the story of five Michigan State students: Ash, Cheryl, Scotty, Linda and Shelly who travel to a cabin in the forest in Tennessee for a weekend of fun and relaxation. Once in the cabin, Cheryl gets hypnotized after watching the pendulum of an old clock swinging back and forth and enters a trance. Her hand draws a deformed demonic face that turns out to be the same image of the *Necronomicon* (a fictional textbook of magic) they find later in the basement next to a tape recorder. The five friends listen to the recordings of a scientist who had visited the cabin before and discovered it was infected with demons. In the recordings there are incantations that release all the supernatural evil forces. Cheryl becomes anxious and after leaving the cabin through the window, she gets raped by some possessed trees. Once she returns, the others don't quite believe her story but Ash agrees to take her back to town. However, the bridge is now broken and they can't leave. Cheryl becomes demonically possessed, and continues to get worse, stabbing Linda with a pencil. The group traps her in the cellar. Soon, Shelly also becomes possessed and attacks Scotty who dismembers her with an axe and buries her outside. Linda also becomes possessed and Ash decapitates her and buries her outside. After returning to the cabin, Ash discovers Cheryl has escaped from the trap. At that moment Ash is attacked by Scotty – who is also possessed – and Cheryl. Ash is able to save his life by burning the *Necronomicon* in the fire, but early that morning he is attacked again.

The musical score combines horror and comedy with majesty; the music and the end credits are reminiscent of a Woody Allen film. It is unclear whether the five friends take some hallucinogenic substance during the dinner or at the moment they arrive in the cabin but the experiences they go through could well be explained by the effects of a bad trip due to ingestion of LSD or hallucinogenic mushrooms. A shared psychotic disorder is characterized by a person becoming delusional and inducing their beliefs in a second person. Influenced by French psychiatric literature, shared psychotic disorder was historically termed *folie à deux* (madness of two). If the ideas can affect more than one person, *folie à pluisire* (madness of many), or "mass hysteria," would be the appropriate term. The experiences of the five students at the cabin include believing that they have been possessed by demons, and hallucinations with catastrophic results are suggestive of a *folie à cinq* or madness of five.

Another case of demonic possession that received great media attention was the case of Anneliese Michel. She was born in 1952 in Bavaria, Germany, and as a teenager she was diagnosed with temporal lobe seizures. She was treated with phenytoin and later with carbamazepine. After high school, she left her hometown to attend university. Her peers described her as someone who was withdrawn from social activities and hyperreligious. During her first year of university she began hearing voices and so began taking antipsychotic medication. Feeling that she was not getting enough help from orthodox medicine, at the age of twenty-three she started receiving exorcisms conducted by two local priests with the approval of her parents. After a few months, she stopped eating and died from malnourishment and dehydration. Following her death, her parents and the two priests were charged with negligence. Her story served as inspiration for two feature films: *The Exorcism of Emily Rose* (2005) by Scott Derrickson, which focuses on the trial after her death, and *Requiem* by Hans Christian-Schmid (2006), which offers a realistic depiction of the events.

In *Requiem*, Michaela (the character inspired by Anneliese Michel) is portrayed as a real case of temporal lobe epilepsy. A typical temporal lobe seizure starts with an aura characterized by a sudden sense of fear, déjà vu, depersonalization, derealization, a strange odor or taste, and misperceptions, following a seizure that may last from thirty seconds to two minutes. It may involve unusual finger movements, behavior arrest, dystonia of the muscles, staring, lip smacking and possible evolvement to convulsions. After the seizure a period of confusion, sleepiness or amnesia may occur. Norman Geschwind wrote extensively on the characteristic personality traits of epilepsy. According to his writings, these include hypergraphia, hyperreligiosity, hyposexuality, and intensified emotional responses and circumstantiality in conversations. Of all these traits, more recent research has found consistent evidence only for hyposexuality, which could be related to abnormalities in the pathways between the temporal lobe and the hypothalamus. Psychotic symptoms such as hallucinations, hearing voices and delusions of a religious and non-religious nature as well as paranoia or body perceptions can be common in epilepsy as well and can happen before and during seizures and at times in seizure-free periods.

Michaela, as portrayed in the film, lives in rural Bavaria in a conservative Catholic family. She has epilepsy and takes medication. After finishing high school, she leaves her town to study at the University of Tübingen. There, she befriends another girl from the same town, Hannah, and starts dating Stefan, a fellow student. Dealing with the stress of adjusting to new school life and after stopping her medication, Michaela begins to experience temporal lobe seizures. She is once discovered sleeping on the floor by Hannah (displaying the characteristic excessive sleepiness after an episode). Michaela asks Hannah to keep her epilepsy problem a secret and not tell her parents; otherwise they may not allow her to continue at the university. In a short period of time, Michaela begins to experience hallucinations and starts to believe that these are related to demonic possession. She visits a local priest and tells him that she was prevented by external forces from touching a rosary. The priest does not believe her at first but later he introduces her to a younger priest who is more open to the idea. In the meantime, Michaela also enjoys the opportunities that university life offers. When she returns home for

Christmas she finds her mother is very cold towards her and throws all her new modern clothes into the trash bin. Throughout the film, Michaela starts to get depressed as she has more seizure episodes and experiences more hallucinations. She agrees to have an electroencephalogram done and to restart seizure medication but her neurologist recommends she also see a psychiatrist for management of her psychotic symptoms. Michaela is hesitant to take up treatment and finally tells her parents that she has been possessed by a number of demons while also showing classical signs of demonic possession (such as rejecting religious objects). Her parents call the priest who manages to have an exorcism approved for Michaela by the local bishop.

In the film we can see how Michaela is certainly struggling and conflicted between her past life and her new one. Psychologically Michaela is a very religious woman guided by superego-related values. Moving to university is revealing but stressful, as she discovers her own sexuality and begins going to parties, and her new life is reflected by her new clothes, something that is immediately disapproved of by her strict mother as soon as she returns home for Christmas. Michaela's epilepsy continues to worsen and medicine does not seem to be much help; in fact, in epilepsy, many patients do not respond well to anticonvulsive medication. (A 60 percent decrease in symptoms and episodes is considered a good response.) For Michaela, demonic possession serves a purpose, an escape from home and avoidance of doctors, and it provides a more acceptable explanation according to her belief system. Her parents and the priests will try to help her. Due to her demonic possession, she won't have to go back to study at Tübingen, something that was probably becoming overwhelming for her.

In 2010, Daniel Stamm directed *The Last Exorcism*, a reality film set in Louisiana, the land where voodoo and Catholicism coexist. Reverend Cotton Marcus is a preacher at Baton Rouge who agrees to participate in a documentary with Iris, the director of the documentary, and Daniel, the cameraman. Marcus reveals that he had a crisis of faith after his son was born sick. Though he does not really believe in the Devil he practices exorcisms for some families to relieve their suffering. His exorcisms are quite peculiar: he adds chemicals to the water to create a sensation of boiling, he has a stereo to reproduce sounds of demons and with cables he can create an illusion of telekinesis in the room. He believes he can help some families who believe in demonic possessions and would otherwise not go to see a medical professional for these kinds of problems. Marcus receives a letter from Louis, a farmer in rural Louisiana who believes his daughter Nell has been possessed. Louis lost his wife to breast cancer a couple years before and had a religious awakening; he decided to home school his children to give them a more fundamentalist Christian education. However, since losing his wife, he also has started drinking more. Marcus performs an exorcism and leaves the house, but that night, Nell runs to their motel seeking help. Nell continues to behave as if there is a problem, acting strangely. She cuts her brother with a knife when he is trying to restrain her and their father has to take him to hospital. The brother writes a note not to leave her with his father, which raises some suspicion of abuse by Louis who has left Nell chained to the bed (according to the New Testament, demoniacs must be restrained with chains). Marcus stays in the house with Nell, Iris and Daniel, and Louis takes his son to the hospital. That night, Nell kills a cat, and later makes a collage depicting Marcus burning while holding a crucifix, Iris being cut into pieces and Daniel being beheaded as a presage of what is going to happen. Daniel begins to fear for his life as Nell is showing some psychopathic behaviors but Marcus manages to keep the situation calm. After several failed attempts to convince Louis to take her to a psychiatrist, Marcus agrees to a second exorcism. In this one, Nell begins speaking in tongues, seems to have an unusual strength, twitches her body and talks with a strong male voice. She claims to be Abalam, a demon traditionally depicted with a strong body and a female face. Nell also reveals that she is pregnant. Louis later returns and asks Marcus for another exorcism. Marcus accuses him of incest but Nell states her son's father is a boy called Logan who works at the local diner. Marcus then believes that Nell's possession has been acting out her pregnancy secret. Now that everyone knows the truth, calmness is restored and they are happy to leave the family in good standing. However, prior to leaving the town they see the diner where Logan works by chance and stop to talk to him for a few minutes. Logan tells them that he is not the father of the child. He is gay and talked to Nell only once. At this point, Marcus decides to return to the house and finds it empty, with Satanic symbols all over the walls. They look for the family outside and find a Satanic ritual led by the local priest, and Nell is delivering a demonic fetal creature that is immediately thrown to the fire while Louis is tied up to a tree. As the fire is getting bigger due to the action of the demon, Marcus runs to it with his crucifix, praying out loud, and dies in the flames; the other members of the sect finish the work according to the foretelling of Nell's collage.

Despite the film's Satanic conclusion, a narrative of child abuse is described. Louis lost his wife to breast cancer, and since then he has been coping by drinking more and by a return to fundamental Christianity. The family has been gradually estranged from social contact with the rest of the people in town. This situation creates a setting for incest and sexual abuse. Under the influence, a lonely, isolated Louis could well have raped his daughter. If Nell gets pregnant to her father, a conflict arises as to how to deal with it. Nell seems unable to report her father, in part due to her own psychological struggles, her strict education and the poor psychosocial environment. In this kind of setting, a demonic possession provides a fitting solution to the problem. Nell acts out her anxiety through the possession and asks for help. Once Reverend Marcus arrives, she unconsciously cues him to the discovery of her pregnancy.

Similarly to Nell's case, in *The Rite* (2011) an exorcist (played by Anthony Hopkins) attempts to release the demons from a woman who has been impregnated by her father. Later she dies of blood loss in the hospital, and the exorcist begins to experience similar signs of demonic possession. In Couvade syndrome, also called sympathetic pregnancy, the partner of a pregnant woman can develop similar symptoms of nausea, weight gain, aches and cravings. In this case the priest was the closest person to the demonically possessed young lady. After her death, frustrated with not having been able to save her, he will show similar symptoms of possession, likely due to either an unconscious need to identify with the victim or punishment for not being able to rescue her.

James Wan is an Australian film director of Malaysian descent who became world famous with the release of his most popular films *Saw* (2004) and *Insidious* (2011). One of his most recent films, *The Conjuring* (2013) was a commercial success and very well received by critics. It is based on the story of the Perron family who after moving to a farmhouse they bought in an auction on Rhode Island gradually discover that it is haunted by a witch who killed her son right before hanging herself. Before doing that, she cursed whoever would take her land in future generations. Ed and Lorraine Warren are two famous demonologists recognized by the Catholic Church, who discover that the spirit has infected Mrs. Perron with the intention of possessing her and killing her youngest daughter. Only an exorcism will be able to save the Perron family. The film uses elements from haunted house, paranormal psychology and demonic possession subgenres. In real life, Ed and Lorraine Warren were in fact two famous demonologists in Connecticut and their cases served as inspiration for major motion films including *The Amityville Horror* (1979, 2005), *The Haunting in Connecticut* (2009), and *Annabelle* (2014). Today, Lorraine Warren still runs the museum of the occult in her house in Monroe, Connecticut. The doll Annabelle is displayed in the exhibit together with other possessed objects. Ralph Sarchie is a retired police officer and demonologist in the Bronx who befriended the Warrens and wrote a book called *Beware the Night*, which inspired the recent motion picture *Deliver Us from Evil* (2014).

CHAPTER 8

The Supernatural

THE TERM "SUPERNATURAL" – above nature – refers to phenomena that are not subject to the laws of nature. In contrast to naturalism, a philosophical approach that embraces the scientific method and rejects existence beyond the laws of physics, supernaturalism entails belief in the otherworldly realm. Supernaturalism has been traditionally related to magical thinking and all forms of religion.

Since the origins of consciousness and self-awareness, humans have attempted to provide explanations for the intrinsic mechanisms of nature. While the first humans likely used magical supernatural explanations for climate and weather changes, the growth of flora, animal reproduction, astrology, and the mystery of life and death, with the rise of science a division between the natural and the supernatural was established. As a result, the field of supernaturalism has been often relegated to faith or odd beliefs beyond what are scientifically understood as the laws of nature. Yet, some scientific fields such as cosmology or quantum mechanics may fall between the two disciplines. An example of it is the popular "string theory" that attempts to explain all the intrinsic mechanisms in the universe and solve the problems of black hole physics, early cosmology, and nuclear physics; it proposes that all objects in the universe are formed by filaments (strings) and membranes (branes) of energy and the existence of several unobservable dimensions.

One of the first supernatural films in Hollywood was *King Kong* (1933). Kong, a giant gorilla, is the king of Skull Island which is plagued by dinosaurs. The film commences in Manhattan. Carl Denham is a famous film director known for his wildlife motion movies. He is desperately looking in the streets of New York for his next movie star. Finally he finds Ann, a beautiful, naïve, penniless blonde woman. He convinces her to join him in an adventure. Ann first thinks the "adventure" might imply sexual favors, but Carl reassures her that that is not the deal. The director and the actress travel in a large ship called *The Venture*. Only Carl knows their final destination. On the ship, Ann is the only woman among all the men and is causing an obvious sexual tension. Jack Driscoll, the first mate, has an apathetic attitude but soon it is hinted that he has an attraction for her.

At some point in their journey, Carl reveals to the crew that they are arriving at Skull Island where they will presumably film their next movie. Once they arrive at the island, they encounter a tribe of men that are ritualistically dancing around a woman prepared for sacrifice. For the humans of Skull Island, magical supernatural explanations are still used to elucidate natural phenomena. Here, this ritual sacrifice intends to control the wrath of Kong. The chief of the tribe tells the crew that the woman in question is "the bride of Kong." However, right after seeing Ann, he attempts to negotiate with the crew an exchange of six of his women for the actress whom he refers as the "golden woman." As expected, the crew does not accept the deal and return to the ship. On the same night, several tribesmen on small boats go to the ship and kidnap the golden woman. They offer her on an altar to their deity. Soon, a giant gorilla arrives and takes her with him into the jungle. Immediately the crew starts a search in the jungle, encountering a number of dinosaurs they have to fight. In the meantime, Kong kills a *Tyrannosaurus* that is trying to attack Ann and later at his lair he protects her from a giant snake. After that, Kong has a moment of intimacy with his new lover. However, the gorilla does not seem to know how to proceed. First he slowly takes off her clothes while cuddling her innocently. At that moment, Jack arrives and taking advantage of Kong's distraction when he is killing a *Pteranodon* that tries to fly away with the golden woman, Jack takes her with him down the cliff to the water. Now Kong tries to rescue his girlfriend back from the white men but they are superior in number and use all their weapons to knock him unconscious. When they are about to leave, Carl has the idea of taking the gorilla with them to Broadway and attempting to profit from the beast.

In the following scene, people are queuing for the expensive Broadway show *Kong, The Eighth Wonder of the World*. After the curtain opens, Carl glamorously introduces the audience to the chained giant gorilla and invites Ann and Jack to come and have photographs taken with "the beast." With the flashes of the journalists, Kong becomes agitated and destroys the steel chains. Ann is whisked to the hotel but Kong finds her one more time and takes her with him. However, the gorilla seems lost in the city; disoriented in the Asphalt Jungle he does not know what to do to or where to go to survive. Desperate, he wrecks an elevated train and in an attempt to find a safe place, he climbs the Empire State Building. Once at the top, he is shot at by four military airplanes. Kong fights them and knocks one down but finally succumbs to the gunfire, but not before managing to secure his beloved bride in a safe place. In the most romantic moment, Kong protects her one more time before falling off the Empire State. Carl says that it was not the airplanes that ended Kong's life but the Beauty that killed the Beast.

In *King Kong*, Ann, the golden woman, represents a sexual bomb. Portrayed as an innocent, highly suggestible and physically astonishing blonde, she causes chaos anywhere she goes. This outcome is already anticipated in the film's opening scene that contains an old Arab proverb stating: "And the Prophet said, 'And lo, the beast looked upon the face of beauty. And it stayed its hand from killing. And from that day, it was as one dead.'" In the presence of the golden woman, men regress to a more animalistic stage driven by their libidos. First at the ship, Jack, the alpha male, controls the other males and finally gets the right to kiss her. Once they get to Skull Island, the chief of the native tribe immediately offers a six for one deal in exchange for the golden woman. Not being able to get her through peaceful negotiation, he orders she be kidnapped. At Skull Island, Kong also falls for her right away and puts his life at risk for her on more than one occasion. First he fights the dinosaurs and finally the airplanes. While Kong allegorically would represent the sexual drives of the id, the dinosaurs would be a harsh superego attempting to violently repress sexual desire. The dinosaurs recognize the danger that she poses for the island's harmony and attempt to exterminate her at first sight.

The golden woman awakens the sexual drives of all the male mammals, no matter their species, or ethnicity, turning them into voracious competitors for the precious gift that she represents. At Skull Island, Kong has a clear advantage and succeeds in protecting her on several occasions. Ann also understands that Kong is her best bet to survive the multiple threats of the jungle and soon stops trying to escape, surrendering to the island's alpha male. However, a problem arises and due to anatomical differences between the giant gorilla and the blonde lady, copulation will not be possible. Object relation theorist and psychoanalyst Melanie Klein states that since birth, the child is conflicted with Eros, or life, drives and Thanatos, or death, drives. In this scene, in which we see the moment of intimacy between the gorilla and the golden woman, the conflict between the Eros and the Thanatos is portrayed. In case of copulation, the gorilla would probably end the golden woman's life due to the size of his giant penis. In contrast, once in Manhattan, the Asphalt Island, Jack becomes the preferred sexual partner. Kong will not be able to survive there and won't know how to protect her. Ann is confused and conflicted by the love of the two pretenders. In the end Kong will have to die so that calm is restored.

Other kinds of animals have also played a role in supernatural films. In *The Birds* (1963) Alfred Hitchcock was inspired by an actual event that took place in the town of Capitola, a summer city in Monterey Bay in California. One morning in 1961, the residents woke up and found a large number of dead sooty shearwater birds slamming on their rooftops and the streets covered with dead birds. News reports stated the birds of the bay had been poisoned with domoic acid from shellfish. Hitchcock immediately thought this story could be the basis for his next film. For that he hired Evan Hunter to write a script adapted from Daphne du Maurier's short story "The Birds."

The film's main character is Melanie Daniels, a young and beautiful social-ite who meets Mitch Brenner, a handsome lawyer, at a San Francisco Bay shop. Intrigued by this encounter, Melanie finds his address in Bodega Bay and goes secretly to deposit a birdcage with a pair of lovebirds and a note at his house. Mitch, however, spots her with his binoculars at the bay and invites her for dinner. Once there, Melanie finds out that Mitch lives with his widowed mother, Lydia. While at the house, the people in town begin to suffer mysterious unexplained bird attacks. The attacks continue to escalate, to the extent that a number of seagulls, crows and other bird species commit murders, and attack the children and everyone in town. There is no clear explanation as to why this is happening. Melanie, Mitch and Lydia will have to escape in order to survive the bird attacks.

The scenes of the birds attempting to enter the house when Mitch is try-ing to seal the doors and the windows have some parallels with the scenes in George Romero's *Night of the Living Dead* in which Ben attempts to seal the house to prevent the zombie attacks. As in zombie films, Hitchcock's *The Birds* portrays an apocalyptic vision of the world.

Slovenian philosopher Slavoj Žižek has an interesting interpretation of Hitchcock's *The Birds* using the psychoanalytic theories of Sigmund Freud and Jacques Lacan. According to Žižek, Melanie arrives in the Bay Area as an intruder who threatens the harmony of the symbolic order. The "symbolic order" is a term used by Jacques Lacan to designate the societal rules and norms a child needs to accept once he or she acquires language to function in society. Mitch and Lydia live in a symbolic incestuous relationship. After Lydia became a widow, Mitch grew up as the man of the house. The sexual tension between the mother and the son is reflected in several scenes. This can be seen as an example of Oedipal victory. The father died and the son took over. Melanie is now an intruder that threatens the sexual harmony in the house. Once Melanie enters the picture, she alters the desire and the symbolic order, distorting reality. In the first attack, we see Melanie, a fantasy object who threatens reality, allowing a bird to attack her. According to Žižek, this is the maternal superego attempting to suppress Mitch's desires for Melanie. This break in reality allows for an intruder, the birds, to enter their world and repress the sexual desire.

It's Alive (1974) is a horror genre B-movie directed by Larry Cohen. Despite the low budget he was able to recruit Bernard Herrmann (*Psycho*, *Vertigo*) for the soundtrack and Rick Baker (*The Exorcist*, *Michael Jackson's Thriller*, *An American Werewolf in London*) for the make-up effects. The story is set in Los Angeles. Frank and his wife Lenore are excited because they are about to have their second child after years of using oral contracep-tion. Unfortunately, Lenore delivers a grossly deformed child with fangs and claws. The gynecologist tries to suffocate him but the baby is able to defend himself, kill the staff at the delivery room and escape. The police get involved in the case, looking for the child. The creature is attempting to return to his parents' home while killing anyone he encounters on his way. In the interim the fertility doctor calls the pharmaceutical company that manufactures the contraceptive pills Lenore took during pregnancy. The executive believes that the pills are likely to be the cause of the fetal malformation and suggests the baby be killed to prevent liability on the company. Frank gives them permission to study the child once he is captured.

At some point, the baby is able to reach his parents' home. Lenore is willing to protect him but when Frank discovers him, he attempts to shoot him but the child escapes and goes to the basement. Frank is about to shoot him again but realizes the child is frightened and feels the urge to protect him. Once the police arrive in the house, Frank begs them to not kill his child. When the fertility doctor urges them to shoot the baby, he leaves his father's arms and attacks the doctor. The police shoot, killing both of them. The same day, it is learnt that another malformed child has been born in Seattle.

An interesting moment in the film is when Frank acknowledges that like Frankenstein he is estranged from the life he has created. The director likely used the name "Frank" for this reason. When the baby is born, Frank shows ambivalent feelings at first but finally states that the creature is not his child. Lenore instead feels much more confused with the situation. The media harasses the couple and Frank, who is a successful public relations man, is laid off work by his boss to prevent the story damaging the image of the company.

As portrayed in the film, families of children with physical deformities or intellectual disabilities tend to suffer from the feeling of burden, decreased quality of life, social isolation and stigmatization. Research shows that once a child is known to have an intellectual disability, the family anticipates social isolation. Frank fails to recognize his baby as his and gives custody of him to the authorities for research purposes.

A central theme is the fear of having a son with deformities, although today many metabolic and genetic disorders that can carry intellectual disability and malformation can be detected during pregnancy. For centuries, the parents would discover at birth if the child was healthy and physically intact or not. Thus, there would be a significant amount of anxiety around the delivery. The likelihood of having a child with deformities used to be much higher in the past. Before it was discovered that lack of folic acid during pregnancy could cause neural tube defects in children, anencephaly (the absence of a major portion of the brain or the skull), spina bifida (failure of the spinal column to close completely), and Chiari malformation (the brain tissue expanding into the spinal canal) were more common. To prevent this, folic acid supplementation in pregnant women is standard care nowadays. Also for centuries the damage caused by alcohol during pregnancy was not understood. Surprisingly, the first research publication on fetal alcohol syndrome was published in *The Lancet* only in 1973. Children of mothers who abuse alcohol during pregnancy can have short height and low weight; growth delay; a small head; intellectual disability and low intelligence; behavior problems and facial physical malformations such as small palpebral fissures, flat midface and short nose, thin upper lip, small mandible or micrognathia, epicanthal folds, ear abnormalities and low nasal bridge. Fetal alcohol syndrome continues to be a problem nowadays. Some researchers suggest that alcohol intake during the first few months of pregnancy (a time in which many women still don't know they are pregnant) could be responsible for children with behavioral problems, low academic performance and atypical attention deficit hyperactivity disorder (ADHD) symptoms that don't improve with the use of stimulants.

Released in 1974 after the thalidomide scandal, *It's Alive* seems related to the anxieties in the population around having a child with drug-induced fetal malformation. In the late 1950s, the pharmaceutical company Chemie Grünenthal released the drug thalidomide. The drug was initially indicated as a relaxant for anxiety, insomnia and gastritis. Later it was found that it could help nausea and morning sickness in pregnant women so it was regularly prescribed for that. Unfortunately, in the late 1950s and early 60s the use of this drug during pregnancy was associated with malformation and failure of development of the limbs, a condition called phocomelia. The drug had not been tested with pregnant animals during the patenting process and therefore the possibility of this side effect was unknown. Around 10,000 babies were born with this physical malformation worldwide and half of them did not survive. In 1961, German pediatrician Widukind Lenz suspected the relationship between thalidomide and the dramatically increased incidence of phocomelia. Further research with pregnant rabbits found evidence of thalidomide causing the birth defects. The executive of the pharmaceutical company gave a public apology for the first time in 2012. While the use of this drug became strictly forbidden for pregnant women, thalidomide, due to its autoimmune effects, was found to be very helpful in the treatment of multiple myeloma – a type of cancer with malignant plasma cells – and leprosy.

Thalidomide was initially thought to be an anticonvulsant agent. Today, anticonvulsants such as carbamazepine, oxcarbazepine and valproic acid are helpful in the treatment of mood disorders. They help achieve mood stability in individuals affected with bipolar disorder. However, these drugs have also been related to facial and cardiac abnormalities and neural tube defects. Lithium, the gold standard treatment in bipolar disorder, has also been related to a type of heart defect called Ebstein's anomaly. As a result, psychiatrists have found the treatment of bipolar disorder in pregnant women very challenging. A number of articles with recommendations have been released in the literature during the last two decades generally showing a preference for the use of the least teratogenic drugs like typical antipsychotics such as haloperidol.

In John Carpenter's *The Fog* (1980) a number of ghost lepers come back to Antonio Bay under the magical effect of a supernatural fog and kill anyone they encounter. These lepers are led by Blake, a wealthy man who wanted to build a colony for lepers nearby in 1880. The ancestor of Father Malone, together with five more men, sank the ship in which they were traveling and used their gold to found the town of Antonio Bay. In the present time, Blake and his crew return to Antonio Bay under a magic fog to seek justice.

Due to its chronicity and relatively benign prognosis, leprosy became highly prevalent in communities throughout history. The earliest medical treatises that survive today such as Egyptian papyrus discuss remedies for the disease. In the Bible there are multiple references to leprosy. For instance, Luke 17:11–19 relates an account in which Jesus healed ten men with leprosy as he was going into a village on the border between Samaria and Galilee. After they asked him for help, he commanded them to go and show themselves to the priests. After doing what he asked, they were cleansed from disease. Of all of them, only one, the Samaritan, went back, throwing himself at Jesus's feet and thanking him. Jesus reflected on the fact that only the foreigner had come back to thank and give praise to God. Though leprosy has been often historically understood as punishment from God for sinful behavior, in the Middle Ages people already had an understanding of the contagious nature of the disease. As a result, lepers were often marginalized and made to live in separate communities, drink from different wells and not walk against the wind. With their clothes they were asked to wear some kind of visible distinction that would alert the community about their status as lepers. Leprosy was highly prevalent all over the world. In 1873 Norwegian physician Gerhard Armauer Hansen pointed out an infectious etiology for the disease. As a result, the disease was renamed Hansen disease in the scientific community. However, it was not until the 1940s that the first effective drug, promin (a sulfone) became available. Today this infection, caused by the bacteria *Mycobacterium leprae*, is treated with a combination of three antibiotics: rifampicin, dapsone and clofazimine. Without treatment, the natural course of the disease involves skin and peripheral nerve infection. This can lead to erythematous lesions and chronic granulomas that can affect the skin of the face, buttock and other areas. The disease can be latent for periods of time and reactivate in acute episodes, which in part will depend on the individual's immunity. The disease causes nerve damage and loss of sensation of temperature and pain. Contrary to literary accounts, people with leprosy don't spontaneously lose body parts. Nonetheless, as in diabetes – a disease also involving peripheral nerve impairment – the loss of pain sensation puts the person at higher risk for ulcers in extremities that go unnoticed and are subject to infection to the extent that they could require limb amputation. In fact, lepers have been historically represented in literature and art with bandages covering extremities that have been partially amputated. From an aesthetic and iconographic point of view, modern zombies – wandering bodies in different states of decomposition – seem related to these artistic depictions of lepers.

In *The Fog*, local radio DJ Stevie Wayne receives a piece of wood that her young son Andy has found at the beach with the inscription "Dane" – the name of Blake's ship. Stevie takes the piece to the lighthouse where she broadcasts and leaves it next to the tape player. Mysteriously, the wood seeps water and turns the player off. After that Stevie hears a voice stating "Six must die." In the meantime, the fog, which travels randomly in the opposite direction to the wind, begins to cover the town. With the fog, a number of half-decomposed bodies with hooks and knives knock on people's doors to kill them violently. The fifth victim is Andy's caregiver. Stevie asks the radio station for help to save her son. Nick and Elizabeth hear the message and arrive in time to save him. Stevie suggests they look for shelter in the town's church. There, Father Malone offers Blake and his crew members the church's golden crucifix, something that restores normality in town. In a different scene, Father Malone wonders why Blake did not kill him and took only five lives instead of six, but he is surprised by the ghost who has come back to take the last life.

Taking a Lacanian approach to *The Fog*, we see how a number of sexual threats from the beginning of the film put the symbolic order of Antonio Bay in danger. The first victims are three local fishermen who fantasize about Stevie as they hear her broadcast. One of them is married but acknowledges that marriage is not the status quo. Nick picks up Elizabeth hitchhiking on the road and they have extramarital intercourse on the first night. The fog comes to their house too but he is saved in the last second. Another victim is Dan, the local weatherman who is making passes at Stevie by phone all the time. This setting creates a space for fantasy breaking into reality in an attempt to repress unacceptable sexual behaviors and restore order.

In 1990, Frank Marshall directed *Arachnophobia*, a film that utilizes our unconscious and collective fear of spiders to provoke a feeling of horror. The film starts with a group of entomologists on an expedition to Venezuela. During a routine trapping of insects, the researchers find two spiders that seem to belong to a new species. One of these spiders escapes and bites the photographer of the crew who almost instantaneously has a seizure and dies from the venom. The spider crawls into the coffin that contains the photographer's body and hitches a ride back to the researchers' hometown, Canaima, California, where family physician Ross Jennings who has a spider phobia has just moved with his family with the intention of starting a practice.

Soon, people who appear completely healthy start to die in Canaima and after the death of the town's other doctor, Jennings and the county coroner Milton Briggs realize that the spider bites are the cause of the mysterious deaths. With the help of Dr. Atherton they realize that the Venezuelan spider plans on taking over its new area by creating reproductive offspring with a domestic house spider at Jennings' barn. The physician will have to overcome his fears to save the world from the dangerous spider plague.

Arachnophobia is considered a specific phobia. A phobia involves an excessive fear of a specific object or situation. The diagnosis requires the development of intense anxiety, even to the point of panic, when exposed to the feared object or situation. Persons with specific phobias may anticipate harm, such as being bitten by a spider, or may panic at the mere thought of losing control, like fainting if exposed to the feared object. These phobias are considered the most common mental disorder among women and the second most common among men only after substance-related disorders. The six-month prevalence rates of specific phobias among women can be rated between 13.6 and 16.1 percent and in men between 5.2 and 6.7 percent. The most common feared objects are insects or animals, storms, heights, illness, injury and death. Though phobia runs in families and is thought to have a genetic component, phobia to loud noises is the only phobia that has been proven to be innate. The other phobias are either learned or become epigenetically manifest, resulting from the subject's interaction with the environment. With phobias, in almost every culture specific phobic agents tend to be recurrent, such as spiders or snakes.

From an evolutionary viewpoint these animals have long been considered poisonous and life threatening. According to the theses of Carl Jung, despite these animals not posing a major threat today, the knowledge about the potential devastating consequences of spider or snake bites could have impacted communities, causing a latent fear in our collective unconscious memories. Culturally, these animals have carried negative connotations throughout history. In the Book of Genesis in the Bible, the Devil manifests in the form of a snake to convince Eve to eat from the tree of wisdom.

Psychoanalysis provided one of the first etiological explanations for phobia. In 1909, Sigmund Freud published a paper describing the "Analysis of Phobia in a Five-year-old Boy." In the previous years, Freud had encouraged his friends and colleagues to take notes on their children's development, including this boy, also known as Little Hans. He had developed a phobia to horses at the age of five years old. His father wrote to Freud thinking that he had excessive castration anxiety and the boy had developed a neurotic equinophobia (fear of horses). According to his father, at the age of four, the boy developed an intense fear of leaving the house after witnessing a carthorse collapsing while pulling a heavy load. Little Hans was at the park with the family's maid and his father thought that the boy's fear of horses could be related to sexual over-excitement caused by his mother's caresses together with a fear of the large penises of horses. Freud did not reject this interpretation but encouraged the father to be more flexible and consider other alternatives, such as Little Hans's anxiety being caused by the arrival of his younger daughter and an inadequately satisfied curiosity about the origin of babies. Freud encouraged Little Hans's father to talk to him about coitus but he was hesitant to do so, something that Freud found frustrating. He finally interpreted Little Hans's equinophobia as the result of the anxiety related to the birth of his little sister, his desire to replace his father and become his mother's sexual partner, and emotional conflicts over masturbation. Little Hans's behavior finally improved after his father provided him with sexual education and the two became closer.

In 1920, behavioral psychologist John B. Watson published the case of Little Albert in the *Journal of Experimental Psychology* as a counterpoint to Freud's theory of phobia. Inspired by Ivan Pavlov's experiments with dogs, Watson had created in Little Albert a phobia to rats and rabbits as a conditioned response experimenting with the animals in his lab at Johns Hopkins University. At first Little Albert showed no fear response when exposed to a rabbit, a monkey, a dog and a rat. After pairing the rat with a loud noise Little Albert developed fear and anxiety when faced with the rat. Watson's hypothesis invoked the traditional stimulus–response model of the conditioned reflex to account for the creation of a phobia, which would be aroused by a naturally frightening stimulus (a loud noise) that occurs contiguously with a second inherently neutral stimulus (the rat). As a result of this connection, especially if the two stimuli are paired, the second stimulus becomes capable of evoking the phobia itself.

In *Arachnophobia*, Dr. Jennings overcomes his fear of spiders by confronting it in real life. A common treatment for specific phobia is exposure therapy. In this method, therapists desensitize patients by using a series of gradual, self-paced exposures to the phobic stimuli, and they teach patients various techniques to deal with anxiety, such as muscle relaxation and deep breathing. In cognitive behavioral therapy, the excessive fear of the phobic agent would be approached as a cognitive distortion. The therapist will use techniques to challenge the patient's distorted perceptions about the feared object to reinforce to the patient that the phobic stimulus is safe.

After the success of vampire teenage movie *The Lost Boys*, Joel Schumacher directed *Flatliners* (1990). The film lies between the natural and the supernatural and tells the story of five medical students who use their scientific knowledge to undergo near death experiences and explore what lies beyond death. One of the first psychiatrists who wrote about near death experiences was Elisabeth Kübler-Ross. Though she has been known in the medical field as the person who described the stages of death and dying (denial, anger, bargain, depression and acceptance) later in her career, she began by gathering information from patients who had been clinically dead. Raymond Moody was another psychiatrist interested in near death experiences, and in 1975 he wrote *Life after Life*. In this book he narrated the experiences of 150 patients who had gone through near death experiences. For him, these narratives could provide proof of the existence of life after death.

More recently, with improvement in cardiac resuscitation techniques, the total number of patients who report near death phenomena has increased significantly. Research has shown that near death experiences are universal and independent of age, gender, ethnicity and nationality. In general, most patients under cardiac arrest and lack of brain activity report no memories of the events. However, a smaller number of patients recall several experiences such as a sense of awareness that one is dying, a feeling of wellbeing and peace, out of body experiences, seeing a light or a tunnel, a life review taking place in front of them, seeing deceased relatives and a conscious return into their bodies.

There is a still a strong debate about the authenticity of near death experiences and whether they provide ipso facto any information about what we can expect when we die. However, basic research on neuronal death could still provide us with some understanding about the phenomenon. For instance, it is known that glutamate and other excitatory amino acids are released with neuronal death. Glutamate and its receptors α-amino-3-hydroxy-5-methyl-4-isoxazolepropionic (AMPA) and N-methyl-D-aspartate (NMDA) have been recently thought to play a significant role in the pathophysiology of schizophrenia and psychotic disorders. As a result we could hypothesize that a massive release of glutamate in the brain could explain the "hallucinatory-like" phenomena of near death experiences. In addition, a release of endorphins could explain the overwhelming pleasant feelings of individuals going through near death experiences. Moreover, the hypoxia that happens during brain death could also explain pleasant feelings. It has been also shown that under transitory hypoxia people can report seeing a light or a tunnel. Though not enough to fully explain the phenomenology of out of body experiences that some people report (being able to describe in detail the rescue scenes, the operating room and so on), in some forms of temporal lobe epilepsy, patients describe seeing themselves from outside the body.

The phenomenology of near death experiences has challenged our theories of consciousness. Consciousness is defined as the mind's awareness of itself with respect to the rest of the world. Within the last two decades, psychiatry has embraced a physicalist model of consciousness in which there is no possible consciousness beyond the brain. Consciousness disappears under a naturally or chemically induced coma. Nonetheless, unlike in dreams, people who have near death experiences report a conscious awareness that one is dying and a decision to return to one's body. This has led to some physicians, such as cardiologist Pim van Lommel, constructing a non-local consciousness theory, which would support a consciousness beyond the physical. If this theory were proved correct, the dualistic model of the mind – the Cartesian model – in contrast to the physicalist model, would become more reasonable.

In contrast to the negative near death experiences portrayed in *Flatliners*, in real life most patients remember these experiences as pleasant. In fact many of the people who undergo near death experiences report losing their fear of dying. Nevertheless, the debate around near death experiences as proof of a conscious life after death will remain unresolved.

Many of the supernatural horror films produced in the last decades are based on novels written by Stephen King. Together with Edgar Alan Poe, H.P. Lovecraft, and Clive Barker, King is considered one of the greatest masters of horror of all time. King was born in Portland, Maine in 1947. When he was two years old his father abandoned the family and King was raised in poverty with his mother who worked as a caregiver for the mentally challenged. As a child he witnessed the death of one of his friends when being struck by a train. Though he has no memory of the event, his family told him that he was speechless and in shock. King found his inspiration to write horror novels after reading an H.P. Lovecraft short story, "The Lurker in the Shadows," that he found in an old attic and which belonged to his father. Perhaps, his interest in writing about horror was a way to reconnect with his own father. As an adolescent he became an avid reader and a fan of the horror comic series *Tales from the Crypt*. After graduating from college, he became a high school teacher and wrote his first novel, *Carrie*. After his mother fell ill with uterine cancer King moved with his family to Southern Maine to spend time with her. During that period, King wrote in the garage of a house they rented and produced his second novel, *Salem's Lot*. King's mother passed just before *Carrie* was published, but his aunt had the time to read his novel. At that time King moved to Boulder, Colorado with his family. There, he wrote his third novel, *The Shining*.

King struggled with alcohol dependence and benzodiazepine, cocaine and marijuana abuse during the late 70s and the 80s. He has no recall of writing his novel *Cujo* (1981) due to being under the influence most of the time. With the help of his wife he was able to recover from addiction and has been sober ever since. *Cujo* was adapted to film by Lewis Teague in 1983. The film begins with a Saint Bernard dog being bitten by a rabid bat after sticking his nose in a cave. Vic and his wife Donna Trenton live with their son Tad, who has a fear of monsters. Vic and Donna are in a marital crisis as Vic has discovered Donna is having an affair with her ex-boyfriend. One day they go to a rural area to have their car repaired and encounter the Saint Bernard dog Cujo. Eventually, the dog is affected by rabies and goes mad, killing his owner and a neighbor. Donna returns with her son for more car repairs and they are also attacked by Cujo. They take shelter in their car. Donna now has to manage to leave the car to avoid dying from dehydration and save her son's life.

As reflected in *Cujo*, a collective fear of rabies is still very present in society. Despite rabies being a very rare disease nowadays, that has not always been the case. Cases of rabies are reported in medical literature as early as 2000 BCE. In Mesopotamia, the Laws of Eshnunna discovered in Baghdad,

Iraq dictate that the owner of a rabid dog has the responsibility of taking preventive measures against bites and if a person dies resulting from the bite of a rabid dog, the owner of the dog will be heavily fined. In ancient Greece, the goddess Artemis was considered to be a healer of rabies. Already in the first century there was some knowledge that the infection was transmitted through saliva. During medieval times, Saint Hubertus' key (Hubertus was the patron of hunters and huntsmen) was used as an amulet for healing wounds resulting from bites of dogs with rabies. The key was also thought to protect dogs against the disease. During the Renaissance many experiments were carried out and new information on the disease was obtained; both were fundamental in opening the way for new findings in the future. The first cases of rabies in the United States were documented in Boston in the eighteenth century; however, the disease spread quickly and widely. At the end of the nineteenth century in France, Louis Pasteur argued against the theory that rabies could appear spontaneously and advocated for a contagious etiology to explain rabies. Furthermore he developed a vaccine to prevent it. Thanks to this vaccine, rabies is today considered a very rare disease. In the United States, there are still rabies reservoirs in wild animals such as foxes, skunks, raccoons and bats. The knowledge of rabies has made a significant impact on vampire and zombie culture and cinema. Both vampires and zombies are converted into monsters after a bite. Zombie expert Max Brooks explains a person can turn into a zombie due to the action of a virus that would be transmitted through saliva with a bite. The virus would hypothetically affect the central nervous system, causing rage or madness. In that sense, the birth of vampire and zombie culture can be understood or approached in part as a result of our collective unconscious fear of rabies.

When a person contracts the rabies virus, the symptoms can initially resemble those of the flu. Therefore, a good clinical history asking about recent bites from wild animals or vaccination status is important for detection of the disease. The person can develop fever, headache, anxiety and agitation and characteristic excessive salivation with difficulty swallowing. In addition, though not always the case, in the literature physicians described fear of water or hydrophobia, which is likely related to the fear of swallowing. Once the disease affects the central nervous system, motor paralysis, delirium and hallucinations are common.

One of the most recent recorded cases of rabies affected an eight-year-old girl, a daughter of farmers in rural California in May 2011. Against prognosis, since the disease is thought to be fatal after neurological symptoms develop, the girl was successfully treated with great supportive care and survived. The details of her case are published on the Centers for Disease Control and Prevention (CDC) website and pose an interesting description of how, with the current advances in supportive medical treatment, the little girl survived a disease that for long would have been considered fatal.

A month before presenting with rabies symptoms, the girl had visited her pediatrician with a complaint of a sore throat and vomiting when taking sotalol, a medication previously prescribed for her supraventricular tachycardia. Over the next few days, she developed swallowing difficulties and could drink only small amounts of liquids, but was able to carry on with daily activities. Three days after her initial visit, she was seen in a local emergency department (ED) for poor oral intake and was given intravenous fluids to treat dehydration. Two days later, she complained of abdominal pain without localization and neck and back pain, and was brought back to the ED, where she was evaluated and discharged home with a presumed viral illness. The next day, she returned for a third time to the ED with complaints of sore throat, generalized weakness and abdominal pain suggestive of appendicitis. On physical examination, she was confused with a pulse of 108 beats per minute, blood pressure of 112/87 mmHg, and temperature of 96.7°F (35.9°C). Head and abdominal computed tomography (CT) were unremarkable. A chest CT scan was only remarkable for left lower lobe atelectasis. Because of respiratory distress and acidosis shown by arterial blood gas analysis, she was intubated and placed on a ventilator. She was given intravenous fluids, ceftriaxone and azithromycin and was transferred to a tertiary-care facility.

On admission to the pediatric intensive care unit, neurological examination revealed bilateral lower extremity weakness. Laboratory testing of peripheral blood drawn showed increased white blood cells. Infectious disease testing was negative for rabies at this time, so physicians could not yet know the cause of the patient's affliction. Analysis of the cerebrospinal fluid (CSF) also revealed increased white blood cells, protein and glucose, which was consistent with brain infection. Over the following days, the patient developed ascending flaccid paralysis, decreased level of consciousness, and fever. Magnetic resonance imaging (MRI) of the brain revealed multiple abnormalities in the brain, including the cortical and subcortical regions as well as the periventricular white matter. Electromyography showed motor polyneuropathy with absence of electrical signals in the distal limb muscles in response to stimulation of the respective motor nerves. The patient was given a short course of different antibiotics – ceftriaxone, levofloxacin and azithromycin – to treat possible bacterial pneumonia and *Mycoplasma pneumoniae* encephalitis and was started on an anticonvulsant, levetiracetam, for seizure prophylaxis.

The California Encephalitis Project at the California Department of Public Health Viral and Rickettsial Disease Laboratory (VRDL) was asked to urgently test for enterovirus and West Nile virus. VRDL suggested testing for rabies, given the compatible clinical syndrome, and subsequently detected immunoglobulin G (IgG) and immunoglobulin M (IgM) rabies virus-specific antibodies in serum by indirect fluorescent antibody (IFA) testing.

With a presumptive diagnosis of rabies, the patient was sedated with ketamine and midazolam and started on amantadine and nimodipine to prevent cerebral artery vasospasm, and fludrocortisone and hypertonic saline to maintain her sodium at a level >140 mmol/L. Neither human rabies immunoglobulin nor rabies vaccine was administered.

During the first week of hospitalization, the patient developed autonomic instability manifested as significant hypertension, which required aggressive supportive treatment. These resolved with repositioning of her central venous catheter. A few days later, the patient moved her head spontaneously. Over the next few days, she moved her head more, then began moving her arms and then her legs. With progressive improvement in her strength, she tolerated extubation and was transferred to the pediatric wards one week later. A month after the beginning of symptoms, she was transferred to the rehabilitation service with residual neurological left foot drop. At discharge she showed no signs of cognitive impairment and was able to walk and perform activities of daily living.

Whether the source of infection was one of the pet cats, one of the animals in the farm or a wild animal was never known. The girl did not recall any animal bite. A family horse had died a year earlier, presumably of colon torsion. The body was exhumed but the brain was not in good state for testing.

According to the CDC, human rabies cases in the United States are rare, with only one to three cases reported annually. Thirty-four cases of human rabies have been diagnosed in the United States since 2003, of which ten cases were found to have contracted infection outside of the United States and its territories. The number of human deaths in the United States attributed to rabies has been steadily declining since the 1970s due to animal control and vaccination programs, modern rabies biologics following exposure, and successful outreach campaigns. Rabies vaccination programs have eliminated domestic dogs as reservoirs of rabies in the United States, although we still see 80 to 100 dogs and over 300 cats with rabies each year, usually infected by wildlife when these domesticated pets are not vaccinated against rabies. While the biggest rabies threat in the world (domestic dogs) has been controlled in the United States, interactions with other rabies reservoir species result in 30,000 to 60,000 Americans being vaccinated against rabies each year. In 2012, Bill Wasik and Monica Murphy published the book *Rabid: A Cultural History of the World's Most Diabolical Virus* in which they warned that as this virus is today being neglected due to the low incidence of cases in developed countries, a new pandemic may take place at some point.

In 1984, Fritz Kiersch directed *Children of the Corn*, based on Stephen

King's short story about a sect of children that sacrifices all the adults in town to avoid the wrath of an Abrahamic god called "He Who Walks Behind The Rows." The sect is founded by a boy preacher named Isaac, who claims to have the privilege to speak directly to this god. The name of the fictional town is Gatlin in Nebraska. The town's economy is based mainly on agriculture and after a year of bad harvest, Isaac and his lieutenant Malachai lead the children in town in a mass killing of all the adults using knives and machetes. Those kids who do not want to join the sect get killed too. Once they turn nineteen years old, adolescents go through ritual sacrifice as no adults are allowed in the cult. Job and Sarah don't want to join the cult but Isaac decides to keep them alive, as Sarah seems to have the gift of premonition through her drawings.

The members of the cult also sacrifice in the cornfields all the adults they encounter on the road. Two of these adults are Vicky and Burt who are traveling through Nebraska to Seattle where Burt has a new job as a physician in the emergency room. The signs on the road are confusing so that travelers end up passing through Gatlin. Once they arrive there, they enter a house in an attempt to make a phone call but discover the city is abandoned and all the phone lines are cut. There they meet Sarah in a house. The members of the cult arrive and capture Vicky while Burt is able to escape with the help of Job who takes him to a shelter his father had once built to escape from a potential communist invasion. Once they bandage his wounds, Burt leaves the shelter to rescue his lover. Meanwhile Malachai has started a mutiny against Isaac who is offered to "He Who Walks Behind The Rows." At the same time, Burt arrives, rescues Vicky and confronts the children about their religious practices. At that moment, a resuscitated Isaac, possessed by the evil god, strangles Malachai. With the help of Job, Burt tries to stop "He Who Walks Behind The Rows" by burning the cornfield.

Despite these dramatic narratives, historically human sacrifices have been generally prohibited in most cultures and regarded as murder. Today, there are some exceptional cases of occult sects that practice ritual murder. Usually these cases involve isolated groups of highly influential people led by a psychotic person. Sometimes these situations are referred to in psychiatry as examples of *folie à pluisire* (madness of many) or shared psychotic disorder. *Children of the Corn* describes well an example of these types of sects. Isaac is the charming preacher who claims to talk directly to the evil god. Malachai is the brute force, the leader of the army. Isaac and Malachai control the followers with fear. Similarly to many other religions, chastity and sexual repression are important values in the film. Here, however, not only the leaders but also the followers are chaste. Once followers reach sexual maturity, they are sacrificed. Adults are perceived as a major threat as they are sexual objects. Therefore, they are brutally killed and sacrificed. If this belief system continues, the sect won't last long, as all the chaste followers eventually would become adult and die. As is likely when Isaac or Malachai become adults, the rules would change towards an acceptance of some kind of sexuality that would guarantee continuity. Perhaps only a few men would be allowed to live as adults for the sake of reproduction and preservation, and perhaps the sacrifices would become symbolic, as in current mainstream religions.

Job and Sarah are the intellectuals of the community; they don't accept the religious teachings and therefore they represent a threat to the integrity of the sect. Malachai thinks they must die, but Isaac wants to keep them alive since he thinks he can make good use of Sarah's gift. Anyone who disagrees with them can be victimized. *Children of the Corn* denounces religious fanaticism. Over the last few centuries, religious fanaticism has led to fear, violence, wars and death. Burt makes a final statement in defense of what according to him should be religion. For him, religion is about love. Unfortunately, historically this opinion has not always been shared by many of our religious leaders.

Ritual sacrifice has been almost a constant throughout history in all cultures and regions in the world. In this sense *Children of the Corn* is related to *King Kong*. In both the practice of ritual sacrifice is shown as a way to allay the wrath of an external force. In ancient Greece and Rome people killed and burned animals on altars to offer to the gods. Pilgrims visiting the Oracle of Delphi offered money and an animal for sacrifice to the god Apollo before getting an answer from the priestess of the temple, the Pythia. In Semitic cultures, ritual sacrifice was and continues to be practiced.

While it is thought that human sacrifice was generally abandoned in Europe during the Iron Age, several examples are given in the Bible. For instance, according to the Book of Genesis, God tested the faith of Abraham by asking him to sacrifice his own son Isaac on an altar. Right before Abraham was about to carry out God's command, an angel stopped him and asked him to sacrifice a ram nearby in the bushes. In the Christian religion, this event is thought to foreshadow God's sacrifice of his own son, Jesus, to save mankind. To date, followers of Christianity symbolically consume the body of Jesus Christ during the ceremony of the Eucharist.

In antiquity, however, there are some narratives that show human sacrifice was still practiced. For instance, Julius Caesar describes human sacrifice by Celtic Druids in his *Commentaries on the Gallic War*. While this is possible, Caesar's accounts of the Gallic War were exaggerated and other things he relates have not been proved by other sources.

Human sacrifice was also a regular practice for Vikings prior to their Christianization. Jewish religious minorities in Christian Europe were falsely accused of practicing ritual murders of Christian children in an alleged attempt to reenact the Passion of Christ. In the modern era, human sacrifice has been a regular practice in the so-called New World. The Mayans offered young individuals to the *cenotes* (natural pits) to please the water god Chaac, while the Aztecs were well known for the extensive number of their human sacrifices. For them, the end of the world could happen every fifty-two years and sacrificing humans could keep Huitzilopochtli – the god of war and the sun – calm. Several conquistadors including Hernán Cortés were witnesses to these events and described how the Aztecs would open the chest of young boys and girls to extract their beating hearts and burn them to offer to the idols. Later, they would cut off the arms and legs for banquets and offer the bodies to the beasts.

French author Michel Houellebecq, in his novel *The Possibility of an Island*, comments on the current disappearance of the Christian religion in Europe. In a science fiction mode, Houellebecq establishes the hypothesis of the belief system being replaced by a new religion called the Elohim religion (derived from the Hebrew name for God). In Houellebecq's novel, unlike in traditional religions, the leaders of the Elohim religion are not divine but scientifically much more advanced and preach the message of overcoming old age and death. Guided by a prophet, the goal of the Elohimites was precisely to stop the decrepitude of the body with a voluntary suicide, and gain eternal life through the perpetual cloning (understood as reincarnation) of every individual who adhered to the sect. Houellebecq graphically compares the strategies of the Elohimites with ancient monotheistic religions. However, the Elohimites prove to be much more successful, since they deny an afterlife by claiming that paradise is on Earth and found through a life of sexual pleasure. In the novel, the Elohimites have two basic ritual practices: preservation of the new adepts' DNA for future reincarnation and suicide once the body can no longer satisfy sexual pleasure.

In 1986, Stephen King released his novel *It*, which four years later was adapted into a three-hour TV film (1990). The performance of Tim Curry (*The Rocky Horror Picture Show*) as the monster clown Pennywise was generally praised by reviewers for capturing the spirit of the monster described by King in his novel.

The film is divided into two parts. The first part is focused on the children's struggles to overcome the malevolent monster. The second part addresses the return of these anxieties and struggles in their adulthood. At the beginning of the film a little girl disappears in the town of Derry, Maine after seeing a scary clown between the clothes hanging on the washing line when playing outside. Mike, a local police officer, suspects there might be a child killer in town but the assassin is not identified. This raises the suspicion of something even worse: the return of Pennywise, the dancing clown. Mike starts calling each one of his childhood friends in Derry to alert them, starting with Bill.

In a flashback image, Bill as a child is playing with his little brother Georgie. Later on, Georgie dies when he encounters the clown Pennywise in a drain after losing his paper boat during a storm. After burying his brother, Bill starts experiencing bloody visions in an old album with pictures of Georgie, but he is the only one who is able to see these things. Adults do not seem to be aware of the clown's mischief.

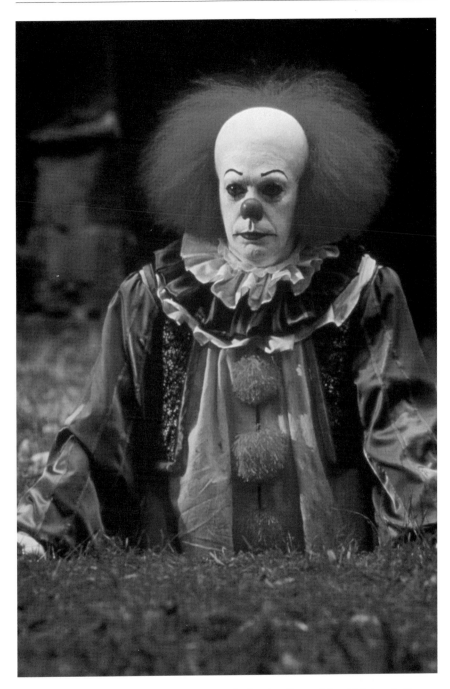

FIGURE 8.1 Pennywise the Clown – the Collective Fear of the Children in the Town of Derry, Maine (*It*) Licensed by Warner Bros. Entertainment Inc. All rights reserved

Soon Bill becomes the group leader of a "club" of outcasts in school. Among them are Eddie, Ben, Richie, Beverly, Stan and Mike. Together they find the strength to confront and get rid of Henry, the local bully who has been abusing each of them on repeated occasions. However, the club will now have to face a major threat, the monster clown Pennywise who has also been bullying each of them separately and taunting them by adopting the form of their biggest fears, such as a werewolf, a mummy and so on.

The different members of the club finally open up to each other about their experiences with the clown. Stan is hesitant to believe it, but he finally accepts the clown's existence. Bill advises his friends that adults won't be able to see the monster because they don't believe in him. The club members decide to counterattack the monster by invoking him with a ritual. Once the clown appears, together they confront him, showing no fear. During the fight, Eddie sprays the eyes of the clown and Beverly fires a slingshot, opening a hole in his head. The kids make the promise that if Pennywise ever comes back to town, they all will have to return to confront him again. Pennywise returns two decades later and now, as adults, all the club members agree to return to Derry to confront their biggest childhood fears.

In *It* there are a number of elements that concern childhood development. Bill, the main character, struggles with a stutter, a type of phonological disorder that usually starts in childhood and can last throughout life. With a stutter, people often have disruptions in the production of speech sounds, also called disfluencies. Often, a stutter can impact social life and daily activities.

For some people, stuttering only happens in specific situations, especially in anxiety-provoking situations such as talking about uncomfortable past experiences; for example, when Bill has to explain to his wife that he has to return to Derry. For other people, however, communication difficulties occur across a number of activities at home, school or work. These people may therefore restrict their social or daily activities, concerned about how others might react to their disfluent speech.

Often, people who struggle with stuttering may develop strategies such as trying to hide their disfluent speech from others by rearranging the words in their sentences, referred to as circumlocution. Other strategies are pretending to forget what they wanted to say, or declining to speak. Overall, the impact of stuttering on daily life can be affected by how the person and others react to the disorder. Stutterers often have comorbid language disorders, and their symptoms can cause significant reactive anxiety. They can benefit from speech and supportive therapies to help them develop strategies to regain a sense of control over their deficits. Bill's stuttering ceases once he becomes an adult. However, when he finds out about the return of Pennywise, he regresses and begins to stutter again when talking to his wife. Furthermore, throughout the film, Bill deals with intense guilt in regards to the death of his little brother Georgie. Perhaps he feels he could have done something to save him by accompanying him during the storm. From a psychiatric perspective, Pennywise the clown could have been a product of his fantasy and imagination to repel and externalize his guilt. By fighting the monster he will be able to undo the tragedy and symbolically remediate the death of his brother. As the leader of the club, he can use his influence to convince his friends about the existence of Pennywise. In that case, a *folie à pluisire* or group hysteria would start among the group members. All of them project their inner fears onto the clown and together they find the strength to confront and fight them, something that results in a therapeutic outcome.

All the club members have been bullied and marginalized. Ben, for instance, is overweight and he has been nicknamed "fat kid" by Henry and his henchmen. Ben is also traumatized by the loss of his father in the Korean War. Pennywise will taunt him, adopting his dad's image. Eddie is a sick child, overprotected by his anxious mother, who puts him in embarrassing situations in front of his friends; he is often taunted by Richie, the joker, who calls him Eddie Spaghetti. Richie is hyperactive; he likely has ADHD, a diagnosis related to a higher capacity for creativity and humor. In fact, children with ADHD are usually told by friends that they are less funny when they are on stimulants. His biggest fear is the wolfman. Beverly lives with her father who is physically abusive. He hits her and unjustly accuses her of inappropriate conduct. In one scene, she runs away from home when he is about to hit her with a belt. Her mother is not in the picture and later on as an adult Beverly will have a lot of difficulty developing good quality intimacy relationships, constantly ending up with abusive boyfriends. Like her father, her boyfriend in adult life is also a narcissistic and sadistic man who hits her and diminishes her all the time. Despite being consciously disapproving of her father's attitude, she unconsciously reproduces that kind of relationship with other men in her adult life. Probably she does not know any better as she never had a positive experience with a male adult. Beverly leaves her boyfriend to join her friends in Derry. We do not get to know for how long she has been abused, but in extreme cases of partner violence, the abused person can develop so-called battered person syndrome. In these clinical scenarios, the abuser releases the tension between the couple with violence and accuses the other person of triggering the situation. The abused person can often feel responsible for being abused and develop symptoms of depression, helplessness and at times experience the whole symptomatology of PTSD with avoidance, re-experiencing, hypervigilance, hyperarousal, and sexual and intimacy issues. Stan seems to be having a harder time accepting the existence of Pennywise, probably because he is the most vulnerable of all. He commits suicide in the bathtub by cutting himself after learning from Mike that the clown is back. The rest of the squad will have to revisit and confront their deeper childhood fears one more time in their adult life.

Pennywise the dancing clown has some similarities with Freddy Krueger.

Both taunt traumatized children when alone and vulnerable. Pennywise talks about appearing in their nightmares. Both Freddy and Pennywise have the same vulnerability: they can be annihilated by confrontation, by being told that people don't believe in them and that they are not scared of them. Also, the frightening clown's jaws quite resemble the ones of the great white shark in Spielberg's classic *Jaws*.

In 1992 Mick Garris directed a film based on Stephen King's novel *Sleepwalkers*. Both the film and novel address the issue of incest, the practice of sexual activity among family members and close relatives. For centuries incest has been a taboo. In most cultures, marriage between close relatives is prohibited and children resulting from incest are considered illegitimate. The strong legal and social disapproval of incest by most societies may be related to empirical observation that children resulting from close family members are at higher risk for diseases that present with physical and mental disability. For example, the high rate of interbreeding among close relatives in royal families or some sectarian religious or ethnic communities has resulted in increased frequency of some rare diseases such as familial Mediterranean fever, Fanconi anemia, Tay–Sachs disease and Gaucher disease. Among the most common genetic diseases cri-du-chat (cry of the cat) syndrome is characterized by a deletion of chromosome 5. This deletion results in cognitive and speech delays, together with feeding problems, a small head and jaw and wide eyes. This condition was first described by French physician Jerome Lejeune in 1963 who named it cri-du-chat due to the characteristic cry of the children affected by this disease which resembles the meowing of a kitten.

Incest among adults and children in families is considered a type of sexual abuse that can lead to psychological trauma, complex forms of PTSD and difficulties with developing psychological maturity. This can make the individual affected by sexual trauma function at a more immature developmental level with patterns of behavior characteristic of the so-called Cluster B personality disorders such as borderline, histrionic, antisocial and narcissistic personality disorder.

In *Sleepwalkers*, Charles Brady is a teenager who lives with his mother Mary who also is his sexual partner. The father is long deceased and the couple, vampires who feed off the life force of virgin women, travel from state to state in search of young female virgins. Despite both having human form, they have the supernatural ability to become invisible and transform into anthropomorphic cats, which is their real nature. In the film, they have just moved to a new town in Indiana where Charles has chosen Tanya, a classmate, as their next victim. Charles seduces Tanya by writing a poem about sleepwalkers and driving her home in his cool car.

Mr. Fallows, the English teacher, begins to investigate Charles after the boy corrects him in front of the other classmates in school. Mr. Fallows is a tedious, narcissistically vulnerable teacher who seeks revenge after that incident.

Fallows, however, discovers that Charles is an impostor who does not come from Ohio as he initially had stated. He follows him on the road and confronts him about that. Charles turns into a demon cat and kills him. Later, Tanya and Charles go on their first date to the cemetery, as Charles shares an interest with Tanya's mom in making tomb engravings and Tanya enjoys photography. Charles attempts to drain her life force when they first kiss. Tanya tries to escape and they engage in a fight in which she plunges a corkscrew into his eye. As this happens, Deputy Sheriff Andy Simpson drives nearby and discovers Charles's car. When Tanya flees to ask him for help, Charles stabs Andy with a pencil in his ear, killing him. After that, the sheriff's cat Clovis attacks Charles. At this point we discover the Achilles tendon of the Sleepwalkers: they seem to be extremely vulnerable to cat attacks. Mortally wounded by Clovis, Charles drives back home to his mother. His mother now goes back to Tanya's house to kidnap her in order to feed her son and save his life. An ailing Charles in the form of a cat tries to drain Tanya's life force one more time but Tanya impedes the process plunging her fingers into his eyes. In the subsequent scene, Clovis leads a group of cats to attack Mary, who bursts into flames.

While in Hitchcock's *The Birds* incest takes place at an unconscious level, *Sleepwalkers* portrays this relationship as a matter of fact. Despite being son and mother, Charles and Mary act as a regular romantic couple. They kiss each other and make romantic statements. They have sexual intercourse on several occasions. From a psychoanalytic viewpoint, this mother–son relationship could allegorically represent an Oedipal victory. The father is long gone and the son has taken the place of the father. Corresponding to a traditional father and head of the family role, Charles is now the provider who hunts young adolescents to feed the family. However, since according to the story Sleepwalkers are an extinct species and the couple has not been able to identify other members of their own kind, this mother and son incestuous relationship might be their best survival bet.

Sleepwalkers are a rare species of human-like cats that feed from virgin adolescents, and are likely to be related to werewolves and vampires. Their vulnerability is to domestic cats, which in this movie are a purifying agent. At the beginning of the film, several pictures of cats as portrayed in ancient Egypt are shown. For Egyptians, the cat was a sacred animal that symbolized fertility. Killing a cat could be punished with death, and cats were purifying animals that helped citizens get rid of rats and plagues. In *Sleepwalkers*, the cats are the counterpoint to the rats in *Nosferatu* or *Salem's Lot*.

Even today, it is quite common to encounter Native American icons when driving on the roads of Maine. One of these icons is the dreamcatcher, which is a net commonly made with a hoop of willow decorated with beads and feathers. According to tradition, dreamcatchers filter negative dreams and allow only positive dreams in the room where the person is sleeping. King's novel *Dreamcatcher* (2001) – not quite based on the Native American tradition – was adapted for film two years later. The story is set in the fictional Derry, Maine in which four outcasts, Henry, Beaver, Jonesy and Pete, acquire special telepathic powers after saving another child with intellectual disability from some bullies. As adults, the four friends have gone their separate ways but have something in common. They all seem to feel miserable. Their slogan is SSDD (Same Shit Different Day). Henry is a psychiatrist who seriously contemplates suicide but he is stopped by his friend's phone call. This year the four friends make it to their annual winter trip to a cabin in the forest. There, they encounter Rick, a confused wandering man, near the cabin. They allow him to stay with them and provide him with warm clothes and water. Rick seems sick and has severe symptoms of dyspepsia and smelly flatulence. A few hours later, as he refuses to leave the bathroom, they have to force the door. Jonesy finds Rick immobile and dead on the toilet, then Rick falls to the side and a lobster-like monstrous creature leaves the toilet and attacks them. In the meantime the army is trying to control an alien invasion. These aliens are sending parasites that use humans as intermediate hosts and may also possess other humans.

The film pays homage to the 1950s alien invasion movies such as *The Thing*, *Invasion of the Body Snatchers* and *Invaders from Mars*. At the same time King portrays his interpretation of the unconscious mind. As in Freudian psychoanalysis, according to the film and novel, the unconscious mind can be accessed through dreams. Jonesy's unconscious mind is divided into several sections like a library. Different memories and thoughts can be retrieved by making conscious efforts to find them. Moreover, Jonesy is possessed by an alien but his true personality also comes out at times. This possession is consistent with the psychiatric theory of dissociative identity. According to this theory, the manifestations of being possessed by an evil force are related to some trauma earlier in the subject's life that was repressed to the unconscious mind and manifests symbolically through this possession. Trauma is still believed to cause dissociative symptoms such as dissociative amnesia, depersonalization, derealization and dissociative identity (formerly double or multiple personality disorder). In dissociative identity, the person unconsciously adopts a new identity that will coexist with the prior identity without being aware of each other. While not explained in the film, the four friends seem depressed in their adult lives as the result of traumatic experiences in their childhood.

The film also addresses a very important issue that concerns psychosomatic medicine and psycho-oncology. Rick has severe gastrointestinal symptoms that make him sick and embarrassed. The diagnosis, however, takes place in the toilet when a significant amount of blood comes out from his anus along with the parasite. Symbolically this represents our fear of suffering a terminal illness such as cancer. Usually we can present unspecific symptoms but the first warning signs take place at the toilet. Identifying blood in our feces can make us very anxious due to the feeling that we may have a serious problem and it is time to go see a doctor. (Nonetheless, most of these cases are associated with hemorrhoids, a relatively benign condition.)

Most human beings understand that they are mortal and at some point in their lives they will eventually face death. Nevertheless, in our current society, death has become a taboo topic. Most humans live with an apparent unawareness of their own mortality. Fear of death is so strong that these thoughts are almost repressed to the unconscious. However, every time we have one of these warning signs (such as rectal blood loss while on the toilet) death anxiety pops up and becomes real. Cancer is perhaps the most feared terminal condition. Though nowadays cancer has a much better prognosis than last century, oncological diseases have been popularly associated with a slow, wasting, deforming and painful unavoidable death. Despite cancer arising from spontaneous mutations in our cells, tumors are generally perceived as foreign objects within our body. In that sense, the alien parasites depicted in *Dreamcatcher* would allegorically represent these tumors or cancers.

Historically, religion has served as a useful method of coping with death anxiety. Nonetheless, in the last few centuries, lay Western society has proposed lay therapies to help patients with cancer cope with their existential anxieties. An example is meaning-centered psychotherapy, a therapy developed by William Breitbart at Memorial Sloan Kettering Cancer Hospital in New York. Breitbart is a child of two Holocaust survivors and developed this therapy inspired by Viktor Frankl's book *Man's Search for Meaning* (1946). Frankl was a Jewish psychiatrist who survived imprisonment in Auschwitz concentration camp and narrated his experiences in this book. According to Frankl, the mind and attitude in every prisoner's life could make an impact on their outcome and survival. Resulting from this, Frankl developed a type of psychotherapy called logotherapy (from the Greek word for meaning). For him, finding meaning in one's life was key to living with satisfaction. While oncologists tend to believe that one's attitude and thinking does not have much impact on the outcome of cancer prognosis (with the exception of smoking cessation, and other healthy lifestyle choices), the techniques proposed by Viktor Frankl can be helpful in the assistance of patients with cancer, especially for those who suffer from irreversible or terminal diseases. Breitbart points out that during the last few weeks or months of life, patients can experience sadness, hopelessness, demoralization and despair to the extent that they may wish to end their lives sooner. Meaning-centered psychotherapy can be helpful to alleviate their existential anxieties. This therapy is divided into seven sessions in which the therapist and the patient discuss in a humanistic way sources of meaning such as one's identity before and after the diagnosis of cancer; the legacy that they have inherited, that they are leaving and that they still can give; and connecting to life through beauty, nature, art and creativity. These techniques can help them find a sense of transcendence, that is to say, a feeling of belonging to something bigger than oneself, and relieve the existential anxiety derived from the knowledge of an eventual death.

Even before directing *The Shawshank Redemption* (1994) and *The Green Mile* (1999), Frank Darabont had an interest in making a movie based on King's novella *The Mist*. Initially the idea was to shoot the film in black and white inspired by Romero's *Night of the Living Dead* but in the end the film was made in color. In fact, Greg Nicotero (make-up artist on *The Day of the Dead*) was commissioned for the creature effects. Years later, Darabont would collaborate again with Nicotero and several of the actors cast in *The Mist* in the popular TV show *The Walking Dead*.

In *The Mist*, scientists at the local army base have opened the door to a new dimension, allowing monster insect-like creatures to enter the real world and kill anyone they encounter without mercy. The invasion occurs while a number of people are at the town's supermarket doing their grocery shopping. One of these characters, Mrs. Carmody, is a religious fanatic who believes the attacks are the beginning of the Armageddon (the battle that according to the Book of Revelation will take place at the end of time). The main characters, David and his son Billy, Amanda, Dan and Irene, manage to escape but discover that the entire town has been destroyed and see no other way out other than suicide.

Suicide is a recurrent topic in *The Mist*. At the supermarket, two soldiers who know the truth about what happened are found hanged in the storage room and at the end of the film, the actors contemplate suicide as they lose hope of escaping from becoming prey of the monsters. Hopelessness is one of the most important single predictors of suicide. In fact prominent psychiatrist Aaron Beck and colleagues found in a study that high scores on the Beck Hopelessness Scale increased the risk of suicide eleven times. In clinical settings, psychiatrists specifically question patients about hopelessness when they report thoughts of suicide at the time that they evaluate for other known risk factors such as prior suicide attempts, a history of substance abuse or mental illness, or other demographic factors such as being male, Caucasian, single, isolated, or unemployed.

While existential philosophy emphasizes the freedom of a person to decide whether to continue or end his or her life, in clinical psychiatry suicide is generally perceived as pathology of the mind that requires treatment even if that means temporarily putting on hold the individual's freedom to make decisions. In the emergency room, patients who present reporting thoughts of suicide are generally evaluated by a psychiatrist who has the power to commit them to a psychiatric unit for their own safety. In fact, in the United States and other Western countries, not committing a patient with suicidal ideation can be considered an act of medical negligence and, therefore, the subject of legal liability.

Despite thorough clinical assessment, evaluation for risk factors and the use of specific comprehensive scales such as the popular Columbia Suicide Severity Rating Scale (C-SSRS) suicide remains difficult to predict. Recently, more attention has been paid to the biological mechanisms of suicide. Similarly to the findings in impulse control disorders and aggression, suicide attempters have been found to have low 5-hydroxyindoleacetic acid (5-HIAA) levels in the CSF. 5-HIAA is a metabolite of serotonin, a neurotransmitter that is thought to have an important role in emotion. In fact many antidepressants' mechanism of action involves an increase of serotonin levels in the brain by selectively inhibiting the reuptake of serotonin in neurons. Today, while researchers continue to attempt to elucidate the role of serotonin abnormalities in suicide, the stress-induced response involving the hypothalamic–pituitary–adrenal (HPA) axis, the locus coeruleus norepinephrine system, the opioid endogen system and the role of inflammation are pieces of the puzzle in the complex neurobiological mechanism of suicide.

In particular, scientists now are trying to decipher the role of inflammation in severe mental illness and suicide. An inflammatory theory of mental illness would imply a systemic approach to the illness. One of the first articles to explain the role of inflammation in mental illness was published in 1947 in the journal *Psychosomatic Medicine*. In the paper, Harry Freeman and Fred Elmadjian found a decreased lymphopenic response to glucose administration in subjects with psychosis versus controls.

Since the discovery of cytokines – proteins secreted by lymphocytes to modulate cell behavior including neurons – the increase of depression and suicide in patients with proinflammatory agents (such as interferon alpha in hepatitis C and interferon beta in multiple sclerosis) and the better understanding of the relationship between the role of inflammation in the modulation of the HPA axis and cortisol, a link between inflammation and suicide has been made. Recent biological research in patients with either suicidal ideation or suicidal attempts shows a relatively specific pattern of cytokine abnormalities in plasma and CSF, more specifically an increase in the levels of interleukin-6 (IL-6) and a decrease in the levels of interleukin-2 (IL-2). At the same time, other studies are paying attention to the existence of specific genetic polymorphisms as well as evidence of inflammation and overexpression of genes that code for inflammatory proteins in the brain tissue of individuals who died by suicide. Inflammation has been seen in areas associated with impulsivity such as the anterior cingular and the dorsolateral prefrontal cortex. In a way, these findings would explain suicide as an impulsive act. People who feel miserable about their lives contemplate suicide as a way to relieve their suffering. Nevertheless, our intrinsic survival instinct, which is probably biologically driven and needed in evolutionary terms for the preservation of our species, interferes with the will to carry out a suicide plan. In moments of extreme despair, or under the influence of substances like alcohol that suppress our executive function capacity, people become more impulsive, increasing the likelihood of suicide. That is probably another reason why imminent suicide becomes so difficult to predict. These biological studies support the existence of a pathophysiological mechanism in the brain of people who have thoughts of suicide, attempted and completed suicide and would support the current medical praxis at least in regards to suicide. Nevertheless neuroscience is still far away from finding specific biomarkers for particular psychiatric phenotypes and even further from solving the enigma of human freedom.

Final Destination by James Wong (2000) brings up the question of causal determinism and fatalism. Following the success of the first film, four more films followed, completing the *Final Destination* franchise. Wong came back one more time to direct the third film of the saga. In the first film, Alex is a superstitious high school student who is getting ready for a trip to Paris with his classmates. The night before the trip he has a nightmare and a premonition that something bad is going to happen, though he cannot really explain what. Once on Flight 180, before take-off, he falls asleep and has a dream about the plane exploding after a catastrophic engine failure, killing everyone on board. After waking up he anxiously tries to alert everyone about the catastrophe and in the altercation that follows, one of his teachers, Valerie, together with his friend Tod and four more students are ordered off the plane – Carter, his girlfriend Terry, Billy and Clear (the only one who also believes Alex's vision). Security does not allow them to return to the plane and they are forced to stay one more day before they can catch the next flight. However, minutes later, while still arguing about what happened, they all witness that Alex's premonition was correct, seeing the plane explode in the air on take-off, killing everyone on board.

The FBI suspects Alex but cannot find proof against him. A few weeks later, the students meet again at the memorial for the classmates they lost in the accident. Alex is estranged and feared by most classmates, as they don't understand how he could have predicted the catastrophe. Only Clear, who was abandoned by her mother and her new boyfriend after her father passed away, is eager to socialize with him. After Tod mysteriously commits suicide in the bathroom, Alex suspects that he and his classmates violated Death's plans and now they are determined to die one way or the other. Alex deciphers Death's design and predicts the pattern in which they will die. He will try to help them beat Death one more time, perhaps with less success.

The film reflects the characteristic survivor's guilt in individuals who survive catastrophes. Often the survivor can feel that they did wrong to survive the event while others did not. Clear and Alex have an interesting relationship. Both of them have problems but of a different nature. Clear was abandoned by her mother after her father and hero passed away accidentally. She feels betrayed by the creator and questions her beliefs. Alex comes from a good supportive family that provided all the nurturing and care he needed. However, he seems to have a more biologically driven problem, which could have been inherited from his father who also has unspecified fears. Alex has bizarre ideas and odd beliefs together with his anxieties. Perhaps he is having the prodromal symptoms of a more serious disorder such as schizophrenia.

Final Destination uses a metaphysical model of causal determinism to explain death and existence. Causal determinism is the philosophical idea that every event is necessitated by antecedents and conditions together with the laws of nature. Alex and his friends violate the laws of nature and escape death. However, Death will take every step to take them back and restore metaphysical harmony. This "Final Destination" that the students are determined to face is consistent with philosophical fatalism, a doctrine that proposes that all events or actions are the result of fate. In that case, humans are determined to not do anything different than what they actually do. All the efforts made by our protagonists to escape death will be useless due to their predetermined and fatalist unavoidable death.

CHAPTER 9

Ghost Hunting and the Paranormal

PARAPSYCHOLOGY IS THE FIELD in psychology that focuses on the study of unexplained phenomena such as telepathy, telekinesis, mind reading, near death experiences, spirit manifestations and apparitions. In the ambit of psychiatry and orthodox psychology, parapsychology has generally been referred to as a pseudo-science. While scientific reproducibility of these phenomena is still yet to be proven, some respected scholars still propose to continue exploring the science behind the paranormal. After all, the world we perceive is limited by our senses.

The paranormal has been long influenced by spiritism, a doctrine founded by Allan Kardec in France during the nineteenth century. In his 1857 book *Le Livre Des Espirits* (The Spirits' Book), he argues that wandering souls and spirits exist and can interact with living people in a positive or in a negative manner depending on whether they are good or bad spirits. With the expansion of spiritism or spiritualism as a religion in England and the United States, a number of people claimed to have special talents that allowed them to communicate with the spirits. These people were known as mediums and soon gained popularity. During the late nineteenth and early twentieth centuries, it was common for séances to be held in the houses of aristocrats and society's upper classes. These sessions usually involved the participation of a medium who would serve as a mediator between the spirits of the deceased and the assistants.

In 1890, Elijah Bond designed a talking board with the alphabet, numbers and the words "yes" and "no" as a tool to facilitate séances. In fact, "ouija" is a made up word from the French *oui* (yes) and German *ja* (yes). The Ouija board became very successful and soon spread. It helped democratize the practice of spiritism among all social classes throughout the twentieth century.

In the field of parapsychology, investigators have more recently used other sophisticated tools for the detection of ghosts, forces and spirits. For example, electromagnetic field meters (EMF meters) can help detect electromagnetic field frequency variations resulting from gamma rays, X-rays, radio waves, ultraviolet rays and so on. Some parapsychologists believe that the measurement of EMF frequencies can help the detection of ghosts. Night vision glasses, audio recorders for the detection of psychophonies (spirits' voices), and thermographic cameras that detect temperature variations can hypothetically suggest the presence of a ghost or spirit in a haunted place. The ability to move objects with the mind (telekinesis) and the ability to perceive different realms in psychosis, and psychedelic themes are other examples of paranormal phenomena.

British cinema features two of the first and most important horror film classics that concern ghosts and the paranormal: *The Innocents* (1961) and *The Haunting* (1963). The first was directed by Jack Clayton and is set in Victorian England. It concerns the story of Miss Giddens as the governess of two apparently lovely children, Miles and Flora. In the first scene, Miss Giddens is hired despite her lack of experience by the children's wealthy uncle as the new governess of the house. The children were orphaned years before and the previous governess had died mysteriously. The uncle is emotionally detached from his niece and nephew and gives Miss Giddens total authority over them. On one of the first days she is taking care of the children, Miss Giddens receives a letter from school informing about Miles's misbehavior with other classmates. Miss Giddens is surprised as both Miles and Flora seem well mannered and sweet kids despite their sometimes concerning behaviors. For example, Miles seems at times flirtatious with Miss Giddens. Once she starts having visions of a man and a woman in the estate, Miss Giddens begins to suspect that the house is haunted and the children are possessed by evil spirits. The governess tells the housekeeper about these visions, and the housekeeper identifies the description as that of the previous governess Miss Jessel and her partner Peter Quint who were often in physical fights and displayed inappropriate sexual behavior in front of the staff and children. Giddens begins to believe that Jessel and Quint's ghosts are possessing the children. She believes the children can potentially be somehow exorcised by revealing their hidden secrets. The children continue to misbehave. One night, Miles tries to kiss her like an adult when she is escorting him to bed. Another day, she sees Jessel at the pond with Flora. Finally Giddens confronts Miles about his odd behavior. Miles confesses he had been obscene and vulgar with the children at the boarding school and at that moment an image of Peter Quint appears behind him. After that Miles collapses and falls unconscious.

Both children show trauma symptoms related to witnessing violence and inappropriate sexual behavior. Miles has more severe symptoms that could be related to sexual abuse. Sexualized behavior, such as kissing adults or using vulgar obscene language with other children or classmates, can be a sign of having been a victim of sexual abuse. A majority of children demonstrate what is considered normal sexualized behavior, which involves some aspects of exploration of their own bodies such as playing "mommies and daddies," "doctors and nurses" and so on. Masturbation during preschool years is also thought appropriate developmentally, and many preschool children touch women's breasts and look at each other's genitalia. However, age-inappropriate sexualized behavior as depicted in *The Innocents* is most commonly seen in sexually abused children, although not in all. These behaviors are usually genitally oriented such as inserting fingers or the penis into a vagina, the anus or oral–genital contact involving a doll, another child or, as in the film, an adult. In these cases, the child can draw penises or genitalia repeatedly, simulating the sexual act and coercing other children. While these behaviors can be seen as a way of reasserting masculinity, they can involve significant problems such as re-experiencing the sexual trauma, suffering social exclusion or in some cases the children can be considered sexual offenders. These behaviors are challenging and at times considered intractable. In the dramatized situation portrayed in *The Innocents*, for Miles death will be the only escape from his imprisoning trauma.

Robert Wise directed *The Haunting* two years after *The Innocents*. Both films have been seen as pioneers in the creation of a new horror film genre of haunted houses and paranormal activity. In the film Hill House was constructed by a wealthy man named Hugh Crain in the nineteenth century, and since its construction both Crain's first and second wife died accidentally in mysterious circumstances. After the deaths Crain's daughter, Abigail, became catatonic and spent the rest of her life in bed with the assistance of a companion. Many years later, the elderly Abigail died while her companion could not assist her; as a result, Abigail's companion committed suicide by hanging.

In the present time, Dr. Markway wants to study paranormal phenomena in the house with the help of a psychic, Theo, and Eleanor, who experienced poltergeist activity as a child. In parallel with Abigail's story, Eleanor spent most of her life caring for her mother, whose recent death has left Eleanor with an intense guilt. One night, Eleanor and Theo hear a supernatural force banging on the door of their dorm. Eleanor believes the house is haunted and is somehow alive. Her mental state deteriorates progressively through the film. She believes everyone is mocking her, and experiences derealization. She cannot tell any more what is real or who is real. Eleanor begins to believe that she is magically falling under the spell of the house as punishment for not providing adequate care for her mother. The group reads a chalk message saying "Help Eleanor come." In the end Eleanor leaves the house in a car, and believing that the car is controlled by a supernatural force, she crashes and dies.

Eleanor certainly could meet criteria for schizophrenia. She experiences hallucinations and delusions, and her behavior becomes erratic and disorganized. In addition she spent most of her life with her mother, isolated and withdrawn. It is unlikely that this would be the first psychotic outbreak; the stress added by the death of her mother – her major life companion – likely influenced this episode. After learning Abigail's companion committed suicide because she could not take care of her, Eleanor begins to rationalize suicide as an escape from her distress. The chalk message was likely written by Eleanor herself consciously or unconsciously.

The closest relation between schizophrenia and the paranormal in a moving picture is probably portrayed in Roman Polanski's *Repulsion* (1965), starring Catherine Deneuve as Carol Ledoux, a Belgian immigrant and manicurist who moves with her older sister Helen to an apartment in Kensington, London. Carol spends most of the day distracted, as if she is in another world. She seems bothered by her sister's boyfriend Michael invading her space at the apartment. Carol's interaction with the opposite gender is bizarre. However, Colin – a friend of the sisters – seems interested in her despite her awkward behavior, but she spurns his advances. Carol's psychic structure continues to disintegrate and she gets distracted at work too. When her sister and her boyfriend go to Italy on a trip, she is left alone at the apartment. At that time her behavior starts to get more bizarre. She leaves a skinned rabbit to rot in the kitchen and begins to hallucinate. First the walls seem to crack, a mysterious man intrudes trying to molest her and hands reach out from the walls to grab her. Due to her severe paranoia she does not even want to leave the house. When Colin breaks into the house to confess his love for her, Carol has to protect herself against the perceived fear.

In Carol's character the incipient phenomenology of a first psychotic outbreak is beautifully portrayed. Etymologically, "psychosis" comes from the Greek word *psyche* (soul) and "-osis" (abnormality). In the medical field, the term "psychosis" is used to refer to a loss of contact with reality. Reality is defined as the state of things as they actually exist, as opposed to fantasy, things or states that are impossible. While a person with psychosis will have impaired reality testing, a person without psychosis would be able to differentiate reality from fiction or imagination. Psychotic symptoms have been classically divided between positive (present in a person with psychosis but not present in those without psychosis) such as delusions, hallucinations, disorganized thinking and behavior, and negative (lacking in a person with psychosis) such as alogia, anhedonia, avolition and affect flattening. Carol seems to have delusional paranoia, that's to say a maintained belief of being persecuted or under threat despite no evidence. She is disgusted by the presence of men. She perceives Colin, an apparently inoffensive object, as a major threat. In the end she begins to experience visual hallucinations, seeing hands reaching out and the walls cracking. These two positive symptoms would be enough to make a diagnosis of schizophrenia. Carol also shows grossly disorganized behavior, as she leaves a rabbit to rot in the kitchen and becomes obsessed with it, and negative symptoms such as lack of spontaneous speech – alogia – social isolation and withdrawal.

Emil Kraepelin was a German psychiatrist whose description of the symptoms of schizophrenia at the end of the nineteenth century continues to be the standard today in clinical practice. Kraepelin, however, coined the term "dementia praecox" – early dementia – to refer to the rapid deteriorating loss of the ability to function. Psychiatrist Eugen Bleuler was the first psychiatrist to use the term "schizophrenia" – split intelligence – to refer to the separation of the psychic structures such as thought, emotion and behavior. In 1911 he wrote *Dementia Praecox oder die Gruppe der Schizophrenien* (Dementia Praecox or the Group of Schizophrenias). For Bleuler, what characterized the diseases were not the florid positive symptoms (delusions, hallucinations, or disorganized thought) but the negative symptoms. Both Kraepelin and Bleuler agreed that positive symptoms could be found in other diseases, such as melancholy or manic-depressive illness. Instead these negative symptoms were more specific to the psychotic disease. For Bleuler "the schizophrenias" were a group of diseases with a common denominator. He argued that schizophrenia could have subtle forms in which the patients were more dysfunctional, saying that the prevalence of the disease was likely higher than previously thought. Bleuler identified the primary symptoms of schizophrenia to develop his theory of internal splits in patients. These symptoms include disturbance in association of thoughts (in which a person's ideas in his or her speech seem disconnected), flattening of affect (lack of expressive emotions), autism (social disconnection), and ambivalence (conflicted attitudes and behaviors). A few decades later Klaus Conrad published *Die beginnende Schizophrenie*, where he described the initial presentation of the disease. From the beginning of *Repulsion*, Carol Ledoux shows all the characteristic prodromal symptoms of a first psychotic episode of schizophrenia: reduced concentration, reduced drive and motivation, anxiety, depressed mood, sleep disturbance, suspiciousness, social withdrawal, irritability and deterioration in role functioning. Furthermore, she seems to have an ambivalent conflict regarding men. Ambivalent thoughts and attitudes towards sexuality can be common in people with psychotic disorders. In Freudian psychoanalysis, paranoia was also viewed as conflicted thoughts about homosexuality. In that case, a paranoid person would be repressing his unacceptable homosexual feelings and projecting them onto another person.

Over the last few decades, researchers have gradually begun to approach psychosis more biologically. Multiple studies have explored the role of blood vessels, genes, infections and antibodies in the pathogenesis of schizophrenia. However, most biological studies have shown little proof of specific biomarkers. Some evidence comes from neuroimaging studies, in which there seems to be agreement that persons with schizophrenia lack the characteristic brain asymmetry. Also, neurophysiological research shows a lack of mismatch negativity – lack of filtering of information by the brain after repeating the same stimulus – in persons with schizophrenia and with prodromal symptoms that end up developing schizophrenia. Scholars are today more inclined to accept a neurodevelopmental rather than neurodegenerative model for the disease. At the same time, there has been increasing evidence of the importance of the social context, culture and country of residence in the prognosis of psychotic illnesses. As in the Carol Ledoux case, schizophrenia seems more prevalent in immigrants and in children of immigrants. For some unexplained reasons, it is hypothesized that the prognosis is better in persons with schizophrenia who reside in developing countries. An explanation for that could be that in some of these countries schizophrenia could be explained in terms of spiritual problems, and as a result people afflicted with schizophrenia would be less stigmatized and are more integrated into the community.

In Western countries, most psychiatrists treat schizophrenia with medication that blocks the dopaminergic (D2) receptors in the brain. Newer antipsychotic receptors also have an action on serotonergic receptors (5HT2A). This blockage of dopaminergic and serotonergic receptors has been shown helpful in the treatment of positive psychotic symptoms. Individuals with schizophrenia have also been shown to have dysregulation of receptors for gamma-aminobutyric acid (GABA), the major inhibitory neurotransmitter. This dysregulation would explain why anxiolytics from the benzodiazepine family (GABA receptor agonists) would alleviate the symptomatology. Today researchers are looking at medications that have an action on the major excitatory neurotransmitter glutamate, such as NMDA receptors, in an attempt to find a somatic treatment for the negative symptoms of schizophrenia. Nonetheless, with the advent of neuroscience, within the last decade an increasing number of papers support a holistic approach in the treatment of psychotic disorders. The role of exercise, physical activity, weight loss, a healthy diet and Omega-3 has been shown to decrease general inflammation and delay grey matter deterioration in the brain significantly. Psychotherapy, for instance, has also been shown to be quite helpful. A study published by Matcheri Keshavan and colleagues showed that cognitive behavioral therapy can prevent grey matter loss of patients with psychotic disorders. This well-balanced biopsychosociocultural model to treat schizophrenia and other mental disorders foresees a good future for the current generation of psychiatrists and their patients.

In 1976 Brian De Palma directed a film based on the first novel by Stephen King, *Carrie*. Before its release, King was initially ambivalent about his novel, and felt that people would not generally be interested in a story based on an adolescent with the power of telekinesis. However, De Palma had read the novel as recommended by a friend of his and became interested. After the success of his previous film *Obsession* (1976) he did not have difficulty finding the budget for the production of *Carrie*.

Carrie is a seventeen-year-old outcast adolescent young girl who lives with her strictly religious and bizarre mother, Margaret. In the first scene, Carrie has her first period while taking a shower at the gym. As she does not know about female menstruation, she gets scared and cries out, with blood on her hands. Her gym classmates immediately begin making fun of her and throw tampons at her instead of trying to help her. Miss Collins, the gym teacher, rescues her and convinces the principal to excuse her from the class. The principal seems unconcerned about Carrie's recent traumatic experiences. No one seems to care about Carrie. As the adolescent arrives home she uses her power of telekinesis to stop a boy on a bicycle from teasing her. This is the first time we learn about her special powers. Once at home, Carrie confronts her mother about not having taught her about menstruation. Carrie's mother seems to be functioning at a psychotic level and believes Carrie has contracted menstruation from sinning.

In the meantime, Miss Collins puts the bullying girls on detention, making them stay extra hours after class doing physical exercises. Chris, the leader of the gang, refuses to participate and as a result she is banned from the prom party. Sue, another girl, feels guilty about Carrie's misfortune and asks her boyfriend Tommy to take Carrie to the prom. Tommy agrees and after a few attempts convinces Carrie to go with him.

While everyone else is getting ready for the prom, Chris schemes with her boyfriend Billy Nolan and best friend Norma to get revenge on Carrie. They go to a farm to slaughter some pigs, drain their blood into a bucket, and place the bucket on one of the rafters in the school gym. Meanwhile, Carrie asks her mother's permission to go to the prom. Instead of supporting her daughter, her mother tells her that Tommy is only after her for sex and that this will lead her down a road to perpetual sin. This leads to a violent argument between Carrie and her mother; Carrie uses her telekinesis to slam windows and doors in her home. After another fight between Carrie and her mother on the night of the prom, Carrie uses her powers to push her mother into a bed and tells her that she must stop worrying.

Carrie and Tommy arrive at the prom, and Carrie begins to feel accepted by Tommy's peers. Miss Collins relates to Carrie the story of her own prom, telling her she should try to keep this beautiful memory forever. Carrie and Tommy dance together; Tommy has since fallen for Carrie and kisses her.

Norma and some of Billy's friends have fixed the ballots so that Carrie and Tommy are elected prom king and queen. When they make their way to the stage, Carrie finally feels accepted by other people. However, this momentary lapse into happiness will soon be spoilt by Chris and her friends who continue with their revenge plan. At that exact moment, Chris yanks the cord, drenching Carrie in pig's blood.

The students gasp and look on in horror. Tommy is furious, but the falling bucket knocks him unconscious. Carrie snaps and imagines that all of the students and faculty are actually laughing at her, something that her mother had warned her would happen. In anger, Carrie uses telekinesis to destroy the gym and kill her peers and teachers, including Miss Collins. When Carrie returns home, she draws a bath. After she has cleaned herself, her mother appears, and tells her she was the result of a strange marital rape. Then, convinced that her daughter is an evil witch, she takes out a chopping knife and stabs Carrie in the back. Carrie falls down the stairs and stumbles away from her mother. When her mother corners her in the kitchen, Carrie uses her power to kill her mother with kitchen knives. After the death, Carrie becomes overwrought with guilt, and using the lit candles, sets her house on fire. The home eventually collapses and Carrie dies among the debris.

Carrie is important to psychiatry as it reflects the issue of child and adolescent bullying in schools. Carrie is a victim of repeated bullying and just when it seems that her suffering is coming to an end, she experiences a type of humiliation that goes beyond imagination. Over the past decade there have been growing concerns about school bullying. Although chronic involvement in bullying is not common, nearly half of the children in schools are thought to have been involved in bullying at some time during childhood. Risk factors that put a person at risk of victimization by bullies can vary from poor social skills or emotional problems to physical factors such as obesity. Being targeted by bullies in school can lead to wide-ranging maladjustment in children.

Perhaps the major masterpiece of psychedelic horror cinema is *Phantasm* (1979). Psychedelia was an artistic movement in the late 60s and 70s influenced by the culture around LSD, a drug designed by Albert Hoffman in Switzerland in 1938 from the parasitic rye fungus *Claviceps purpurea*. LSD typically induces euphoria; enhances capacity of introspection; and alters perception causing pseudo-hallucinations, dream-like states and synesthesia – that's to say the stimulation of a neurological pathway resulting from the stimulation of a different one (e.g. music causing visual perceptions). During the 1950s, the CIA started a secret project called MKULTRA to explore the potential mind-controlling properties of this drug. One of the volunteer participants in the study was Ken Kesey who based on his experiences of meeting patients with psychiatric illnesses in the study wrote the popular novel and later major film *One Flew over the Cuckoo's Nest*. Psychiatrists began researching the properties of LSD in mood and anxiety disorders, substance abuse, hypnosis and psychotherapy. The drug was soon marketed free in San Francisco by Owsley Stanley after Sanz Laboratories lost the patent. Ken Kesey was living in San Francisco and began organizing the so-called Electric Cool Acid parties, where people would gather to take LSD and go on a trip together.

Psychedelia influenced the music scene, with Jefferson Airplane, Cream, The Grateful Dead and Janis Joplin being the prominent leaders in the Bay Area. Psychedelia also had an impact on the arts (as reflected in the famous rock 'n' roll posters by Victor Moscoso and Wes Wilson to mention some examples) and cinema. *The Trip* (1967), *Psych Out* (1968) and *Easy Rider* (1969) are examples of this early psychedelic cinema. Almost a decade later

Phantasm saw light in the theater. The film, directed by Don Coscarelli, starts with Tommy being stabbed by a woman with whom he is having sex at the cemetery. Jody and his friend Reggie attend Tommy's funeral at a funeral home. Jody also takes care of his younger teenage brother Mike as the brothers' parents had died in an accident years before. Mike snoops around the cemetery and sees the mortician known as The Tall Man carrying Tommy's coffin alone. Mike breaks into the mortuary to investigate the mystery and is attacked by a flying sphere that protects the location. When chased by The Tall Man, he cuts his finger and goes home to show it to Jody and convince him that there is something dark going on. Jody, Reggie and Mike discover that The Tall Man is from outer space and is transforming dead bodies into dwarfs to work as slaves in his world. The film's music, slow mode cinematographic scenes and sound effects are congruent with the effects of psychedelic drugs and their impact on the artistic movement based on them.

Considered one of the top masterpieces in horror cinema, Stanley Kubrick's *The Shining* (1980) portrays how unexplained paranormal forces in an isolated hotel can take a person to a total detachment from reality. After the success of Stephen King's novel adaptations of *Carrie* (1976) and *Salem's Lot* (1979), King's third novel centered on the story of a family that moved to the Overlook Hotel in Colorado. Stephen King himself had moved away from Maine in 1974 to live with his wife in Boulder, Colorado for a year. As they arrived they happened to stay one night alone in the Stanley Hotel as the season was closing. That night they were the only guests in Room 217, which was said to be haunted. Three years later his novel *The Shining* was released and soon became commercially successful. Stanley Kubrick was determined to make a horror movie after his historical masterpiece *Barry Lyndon*. Prior to that he had read several of King's novels and thought *The Shining* the most appealing. Although the Stanley Hotel, named the Overlook Hotel for the novel and film, is still standing and welcomes visitors, most of the filming of Kubrick's 1980 movie took place in studios in Great Britain. Nevertheless, the interior was inspired by the Ahwahnee Hotel in Yosemite National Park. The opening shots were filmed at Montana's Glacier National Park. *The Shining*'s cinematography is very innovative and nears perfection with its long shots of slow scenes with wide angles. Krzysztof Penderecki, whose involvement in *The Exorcist* had gained him a reputation, was commissioned for most of the music. Among others, a piece by Bela Bartok conducted by Herbert von Karanjan was also used. The soundtrack provokes a feeling of angst that is beyond control; the choirs create a feeling of being under the influence of some kind of Satanic witchcraft sect or cult.

The Shining has been approached sociologically from different angles. It has been suggested that Kubrick had the conscious or unconscious intention to depict and denounce the Native American Massacre in the United States and the Holocaust. The documentary *Room 237* (2012) discusses this type of symbolism as well as other hypotheses such as Kubrick's attempt to communicate that he had shot the moon landing or hidden symbolism of the Greek Minotaur in one of the posters (a concept linked to the famous labyrinth of the Overlook Hotel).

The story of *The Shining* is centered on the Torrance family. Jack, the father, is a recovering alcoholic who gets a new job as caretaker at the Overlook Hotel during the winter. It sounds like the perfect opportunity for a peaceful time in which to write his upcoming novel. Jack moves to the hotel with his wife Wendy and their son Danny who sees a therapist, as he seems to be dealing with some psychological struggles. Wendy reveals to the therapist that Jack used to have an alcohol problem and on one occasion he ended up hurting Danny after a binge. Danny has an imaginary friend, Tony, who communicates through his finger.

As the family move from Boulder to the Overlook Hotel, the manager advises Jack that the previous person on the job, Charles Grady, had some kind of mental breakdown and ended up killing his family with an axe. Danny had a premonition of the dangers of moving there and has a vision of the elevators flooded with blood. Before leaving the family in the hotel, the chef Dick Hallorann shares with Danny that, like him, he has telepathic and extrasensorial powers. Hallorann tells Danny that he can go anywhere in the hotel but Room 237. Soon, Danny has another vision of two female twins who want to play with him.

During the following weeks, Jack works on his novel but begins to have some concerning behavioral changes. His work on the novel is not advancing and he has a nightmare in which he was killing his family. He relapses on alcohol and begins to experience auditory and visual hallucinations. He talks to the "bartender" at the party hall, Lloyd, and shares with him his frustrations with his wife. He believes she is not being helpful as she does not give him time and space to concentrate on his work. In the bathroom, he has a vision of the previous caretaker, Charles Grady, who alerts him to watch out for his wife, as she might want to leave the hotel, and for Hallorann who might try to help with that. Grady advises Jack to give them some discipline. Danny seems to be deteriorating mentally while Jack and Wendy have an argument about their differences on how to educate him. Later, Wendy finds some bruises on Danny's neck. Wendy accuses Jack but Danny states that he was strangled by a woman in Room 237. Jack goes there and finds a naked young good-looking woman who after kissing him turns into a putrid old lady. Jack's mental state continues to deteriorate in parallel with his heavy drinking. Wendy finds Jack's novel and discovers that he has not been able to write anything other than hundreds of pages with the phrase "All work and no play makes Jack a dull boy." Danny now starts to communicate only through his imaginary friend Tony and addresses his mother as Mrs. Torrance; he seems to have some convulsions and foaming of the mouth. Hallorann has a premonition that there's something terrible happening in the hotel and takes a flight from Florida to Colorado. As he arrives at the hotel, Jack kills him with an axe. After that, a crazed Jack looks for Wendy and Danny but they manage to escape. In the final scene, the audience can see Jack's frozen body in the labyrinth of the hotel.

The film has several elements of interest for psychiatric discussion. The story has been often described as an example of cabin fever: a psychological reaction of anger, anxiety or irritability when a person or a small group of people face prolonged isolation. Nevertheless, when the psychology of each of the characters is analyzed, a rich range of psychopathological traits can be appreciated.

Danny has an imaginary friend, Tony. While imaginary friends are fairly common in developing children, for him it allows relief of his anxieties. Danny has premonitions and visions and at some point goes through a state of altered consciousness with automatisms and foaming from his mouth. All these symptoms are compatible with the phenomenological description of complex partial seizures in temporal lobe epilepsy. The double vision of the twin girls further supports the theory. Furthermore, Danny seems to struggle with anxiety and depressive symptoms as well as impairment of social interaction, something common in children with epilepsy as well as dyslexia, a condition in which it can be easier to read, spell or write from right to left – in one scene he writes REDRUM instead of MURDER during a vision of what could happen to them. In addition, his father has an alcohol problem and at some point became abusive.

Wendy seems to have baseline anxiety but overall is presented as the healthiest one in the family. She seems appropriately concerned for her son and is trying to keep the family together. She supports Jack in his decision to move to the Overlook Hotel and takes care of Danny while Jack works on his novel. However, as she sees her husband's mental health deteriorating to a dangerous level, she has an anxiety breakdown with overwhelming panic and visual hallucinations. She has a vision of Charles Grady with another man dressed like an animal and with a naked butt. This scene has been referred to as a reference to homosexuality. From an analytical perspective, we could hypothesize that this vision is a manifestation of her fear that Jack is homosexual, something that could explain her marital problems. Wendy's case has been described as an example of hysteria. Though the term "hysteria" is no longer used in the realms of modern psychiatry, historically hysteria involved symptoms of emotional excessiveness and visual hallucinations, traits seen in Wendy's character. Using current psychiatric nomenclature, Wendy could well meet criteria for anxiety disorder and conversion disorder, a disorder that involves pseudoneurological symptoms such as visual hallucinations.

Jack has a history of alcoholism. His character was inspired by Stephen King's own struggles with alcohol. As he relapses, he begins to have paranoia and visual and auditory hallucinations of Lloyd and Charles Grady who alert him to the dangers of his wife and Hallorann. His behavior and thinking gradually become disorganized. He neglects his self-care, and seems disheveled. His thought process becomes concrete and ruminative; the only thing he can write is the same sentence over and over. His paranoid delusions, his auditory and visual hallucinations, his disorganized thought and behavior and his negative symptoms fit criteria for a psychotic episode. In psychiatry, a person with two psychotic symptoms for more than a month, or less if treated, can be diagnosed with schizophrenia. However, the term "brief psychotic disorder" is preferred when the symptoms last for less than a month and "schizophreniform disorder" if less than six months. If the disease lasts more than six months a diagnosis of schizophrenia is suggested unless the symptoms are caused by the use of substances, medications or another medical condition. Schizophrenia symptoms usually appear at a younger age, between seventeen and thirty-five years old. In Jack's case, there is no evidence of prior psychotic breakdown suggested in the film. His psychosis becomes manifest as he relapses on alcohol. Therefore, a diagnosis of alcohol-induced psychosis would be the most reasonable one.

The final scene showing the photograph of Jack at the 1921 July 4 party of the Overlook Hotel will remain a mystery that enhances Kubrick's myth and greatness.

Another aspect of the paranormal is a *poltergeist*, a German word used to describe a noisy spirit capable of moving objects in the house and even touching or hitting the persons inhabiting the house. Co-written by Steven Spielberg and directed by Tobe Hooper, who had achieved fame after the release of *The Texas Chainsaw Massacre* (1974), *Poltergeist* (1982) tells the story of the Freelings, a middle-class family who move to a dream house in a suburban area. The father, Steven, is a successful real estate developer and his wife Diane takes care of their three children, Dana, Robbie and Carol Anne, and the dog. Carol Anne, the youngest daughter, and the dog are the first to notice the presence of the supernatural in the house. Diane witnesses telekinesis in the kitchen, and after an earthquake in the house, Carol Anne alerts the family that "they are here." The poltergeist can communicate directly with the girl through the TV when transmitting a white noise image. Soon, Robbie begins to suffer from the evil spirits too. His clown doll becomes possessed and the tree in the yard breaks through window, grabbing him to distract his parents while sucking Carol Anne into the closet. The family realizes that Carol Anne can still communicate with them but she is now in a new dimension. A group of parapsychologists from UC Irvine are able to detect with their equipment the presence of multiple spirits from different people in the house. They alert them that the spirit that is holding Carol Anne could be very dangerous and agree to call an expert psychic medium, Tangina, to assist them in the rescue of their daughter. With the help of Tangina's extrasensorial

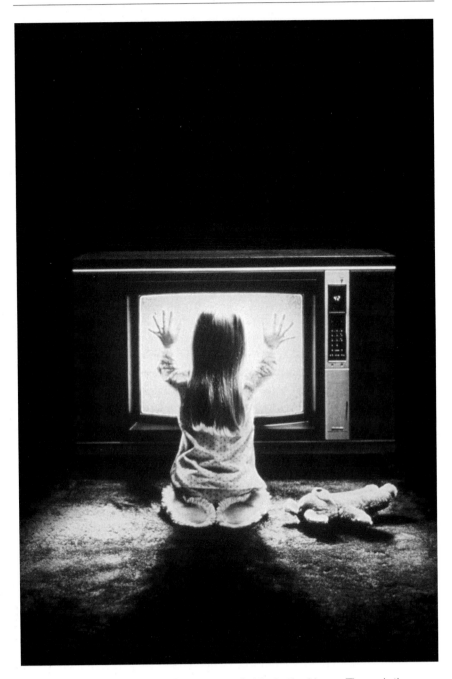

FIGURE 9.1 Little Carol Anne Senses the Spirits in the House Through the Television (*Poltergeist*) Licensed by Warner Bros. Entertainment Inc. All rights reserved

powers they come to the realization that the spirits in the house are not at rest and are distracted by Carol Anne's "light." However, a demon spirit known as The Beast is using Carol Anne to manipulate them as he pleases. Tangina and the rest of the parapsychologists reopen the gate to the dimension where Carol Anne is residing and her mother is able to enter with a rope, rescue her and exit through another door they opened on the ceiling of the living room. Tangina believes the house is now free of spirits. The family plans to move out, but that night the clown doll attacks Robbie again and The Beast attempts to kidnap Carol Anne one more time. Diane is able to take her children outside but falls into a shaft and is harassed by a number of rotten corpses that are rising from their tombs. Steven realizes that his boss had moved the stones but did not move the coffins when relocating the cemetery in order to build in the area and so confronts him. After that the house magically disappears and the spirits now will rest in peace. The Freelings finally move out to a safer place.

Several elements in *Poltergeist* are of interest. The film portrays the characteristic fears of childhood, a fear of certain dolls at night, a fear of a monster or spirit in the closet, and a fear of the tree by the window. Developmentally, Carol Anne is around six years of age and is the first in the family to be able to communicate with the poltergeist. In horror films, in general the younger children between two and seven years of age become aware of these things well before the adults. According to Jean Piaget's stages of development, children of this age would be at the preoperational stage. During this stage children begin to form memory and imagination but their thinking is intuitive and still not logical; they tend to think magically. After this stage, they move towards the concrete operational stage in which they gradually develop logical thinking but their thought process is still concrete. Finally, after eleven years of age, in the formal operational stage, adolescents develop abstract thinking.

While for toddlers and young children magical thinking is the norm, in adult life this way of thinking is rare and at times considered pathological. For instance, in schizotypal personality disorder magical thinking and odd beliefs such as clairvoyance, telepathy, superstition, and the feeling of having a "sixth sense"; bizarre fantasies; and preoccupations are common. Often people with schizotypal personality dress and appear eccentrically and are perceived as odd, which can impair their relationships. Tangina, the medium of the poltergeist, is portrayed as a person with traits of schizotypal personality. In these cases, becoming a psychic reader, a medium, a shaman, or a miraculous healer can be adaptive or resilient. Schizotypal personality traits are frequent in family members of individuals with schizophrenia.

Released the same year as *Poltergeist, The Entity* (1982) tells the story of a woman who claims to be raped every night by a supernatural force, an experience that could psychiatrically be explained by an unconscious trauma pushing towards awareness.

Pet Sematary (1989) is another film adapted from a novel by Stephen King that deals with ghosts and the afterlife. In 1978, Stephen King moved back to a house in his home state to teach at the University of Maine. The house was near a road that was claimed to have taken the life of many pets. As a result, the neighborhood children had created a pet cemetery nearby in the field. Later King's daughter's cat was killed on the road and his son was almost hit one time. Based on his experiences, he wrote the novel *Pet Sematary* and the script of the 1989 film of the same name directed by Mary Lambert. The film was mainly shot at a house on Point Road in Hancock and the cemetery of Bangor in Maine. The area has a lot of forest, small roads and many trucks. For the film, The Ramones wrote the song "Pet Sematary" that was also included on their album *Brain Drain*.

In the film, Louis Creed, a doctor from Chicago, moves with his wife Rachel, his daughter Ellie and her cat Church, and his son Gage to a suburban area somewhere in Lobsterland, Maine. The neighbor Jud advises the family of the dangers of the road. On his first day of work Louis tries to help Victor, a boy who dies soon after due to a traumatic brain injury received in a car accident. Victor manifests in his dreams later and advises him of the dangers of a Native American burial site in the area. One day, Jud takes the family to a pet cemetery (misspelled "sematary" by the children) in the field, where all the pets hit on the road have been buried for decades. Jud shows Ellie the resting place of his own dog, which scares her a little. Ellie begins to struggle with her fears of abandonment as she starts to understand the universality of mortality and the irreversibility of death (something common in early adolescence). She asks her father what his thoughts are about death and dying and life after death as she realizes that her beloved cat, Church, will die one day. That night, Rachel shares with Louis her own fears about death and dying which are related to the fact that she was left alone in the basement when her sister Zelda was dying from spinal meningitis. She struggles with overwhelming feelings of guilt as she felt that her parents had her in the basement because they seemed embarrassed by her. Louis comforts her and offers her a Valium. This type of guilt can also occur in family members of patients who die of cancer. As they see their loved one suffering, they get ambivalent feelings of wanting their suffering to be over and, after they pass away, struggle with guilty feelings about it.

The family's assistant, Missy Dandridge, suffers from chronic stomachaches and, feeling she will never get better, hangs herself. The family goes back to Chicago for Thanksgiving but Louis decides to stay; he grew up an orphan and has an estranged relationship with Rachel's narcissistic and difficult father. During their absence, Church is hit on the road. Jud, realizing that it will be too hard on Ellie, introduces Louis to the same Native American burial site that Victor had warned him about in his dream and advises him to bury Church there. Church shows up the next day in the house but he is now rather aggressive. When the family returns, Ellie realizes Church is more detached and smelly and wonders what happened.

One sunny day in summer, the family is having a picnic outside and Louis teaches Gage how to fly a kite. In a moment of distraction, Gage follows the kite to the road and gets hit by a truck. Rachel's father accuses Louis of the tragedy at the funeral. The family leaves for Chicago for a few days and Louis is left alone in the house. Jud, fearing that he may try to take Gage to the Native American site, goes to visit him and advises him not to do it. Louis does not listen and in an attempt to revive his son, reburies him at the magical site. Ellie has a premonition that something terrible is going to happen and Rachel flies back to Boston and drives back home feeling the same way. In the meantime, Gage has returned, and after grabbing Louis' surgical knife goes and kills Jud at his house. As Rachel arrives at the house, she finds Gage who kills her after she has given him a hug. When Louis finds out what has happened, he puts Gage to sleep with an injection. Despite Victor's warning, he buries Rachel at the ritual ground hoping that, as her death is very recent, the outcome will be better. A zombie-looking Rachel appears in the kitchen the next morning. Louis happily kisses her but she grabs a knife and the scene closes with a scream.

The film beautifully depicts a child's anxiety (Ellie's) when understanding the universality of death and the impaired thinking a person can have right before committing suicide. Missy Dandridge has chronic pain but never asks for help, even when Louis offers to examine her. She may have some distorted cognitions of helplessness and hopelessness. Her communication skills and coping mechanisms are limited. After writing in a letter that she will never feel better, she looks for the quickest and easiest way to solve the problem. In psychiatry, suicide has often been described as an example of short term reward behavior. Instead of asking for help and getting treatment, a person may opt for the shortest path out of their suffering.

Rachel's experiences with her sister Zelda reflect the guilt people often feel when they lose a family member to a chronic deteriorating illness that involves suffering. Moreover, the film portrays the acute stages of grief when losing a loved one, something that involves profound sadness, hopelessness, helplessness, anxiety and emotional lability. The film's take-home point could be to avoid defying the laws of nature. As Jud thoughtfully points out, "Sometimes, dead is better."

Clive Barker's short story "The Forbidden" was adapted to the big screen as the film *Candyman* (1992), directed by Bernard Rose. The movie's story sprang from the urban legend that a hook-handed person named Candyman will appear and kill you if you say his name five times while looking in the mirror and turning the lights off. The legend goes back to the Civil War, in which the son of a former African American slave who became very wealthy from a shoe business grew up an artist in high society and fell in love with the beautiful daughter of a Caucasian man. Enraged by racist feelings, the father hired some people to cut off his son's hand, cover him with honey and let him be stung to death by bees.

In *Candyman*, in Chicago, graduate student Helen becomes interested in a murder at the projects, as rumor says that it could have been perpetrated by Candyman. There, she meets Anne-Marie, one of the residents, a hard-working mother of a newborn, and Jake, a boy who shows them a public bathroom in which a child had allegedly been castrated by the hooked spirit. Helen is attacked by some gang members in the public bathroom. Later in the film, Helen mysteriously wakes up in Anne-Marie's house where her dog has been decapitated and her baby is missing. Anne-Marie is arrested by the police and sent to a forensic psychiatric hospital. There, Candyman kills the psychiatrist and allows Anne-Marie to escape. Helen discovers in some paintings of Candyman at the projects that she looks exactly like his former lover. Candyman is trying to take her with him to his world with the baby. A group of superstitious neighbors at the projects are trying to set a fire to prevent the dangers of Candyman but Helen discovers that the baby is within the trash about to be burnt. She manages to rescue the baby before she dies and prevent Candyman's plans. However, she is cursed with the same fate as Candyman. Later, her cheating boyfriend is at the mirror sighing Helen's name, which after turning off the lights provokes her appearance with revengeful intention.

Interestingly, the *Candyman* movie has some parallels with 1932's *The Mummy*. In both, an unacceptable love has fatal consequences and the spirit is brought back with some kind of ritual to take revenge for a lost love in the present time on a person who physically resembles the former one. With some elements of body horror, the film depicts common childhood and adolescent fears of urban legends. It is almost a universal thing in the collective unconscious of most communities to believe in curses or spells that still threaten communities. The film also portrays the issue of social classes, the aftermath of slavery and community trauma.

From a child and adolescent psychology point of view, *The Sixth Sense* might depict the best example of good and healthy relationship between a patient and a therapist. The film was written and directed by M. Night Shyamalan in 1999 and very soon became a hit. It portrays the story of Dr. Malcolm Crowe, a prominent psychologist who has been awarded by the city of Philadelphia for his work helping children. The night of the award dinner, Malcolm comes back home with his wife Anna, and finds in the bathroom an adult person named Vincent he had treated as a child. After blaming him for his misery, Vincent shoots Malcolm in the stomach before shooting himself in the head.

In the following scene, Malcolm is waiting in the street to meet for the first time his new patient, nine-year-old Cole. Cole seems shy and runs away from Malcolm when he sees him but he is able to talk to him in a church where he is hiding and an empathic relationship between the two commences. Cole seems to be distressed by something Malcolm still has not yet understood. He is lonely, has no friends and is perceived as awkward by his peers. His father is not in the picture and his mother tries to combine work with taking care of him the best way she can after Cole's grandma passed away. In the meantime, the relationship between Malcolm and Anna seems to have deteriorated significantly since the incident with Vincent. The spectator can observe that there is no communication between them.

One day Cole goes with his mother to a birthday party where he is locked in a wardrobe by a couple of bullies and after crying hysterically, his mother rescues him and takes him to the hospital in shock. There, Malcolm visits him and Cole reveals his secret: he sees dead people, all the time. They don't know they're dead and they hear what they want to hear. Malcolm believes Cole is much sicker than he initially thought and could suffer from childhood schizophrenia, but as he continues to examine him and hears an old tape he had from Vincent's case he comes to the realization that both Vincent and Cole have the same kind of extrasensorial ability. This time he is committed to helping him and advises Cole to talk to the deceased people he sees to find out if there is something he can do for them. Cole follows his advice and talks to a little girl who died from poisoning. The girl guides him to a videocassette that captures how her stepmother had poisoned her. Cole gives the videocassette to his father at her funeral and the truth comes out. As he continues to help other dead people, one day, stuck in traffic by an accident, Cole tells his mother his secret and informs her that her own mother is very proud of her every day. Cole seems to be doing much better and Malcolm visits him one more time to close the therapy with a good resolution. Before he leaves, Cole advises him to talk to his wife in dreams. That night, Malcolm talks to her and realizes that he died the day of the award dinner after Vincent shot him and understands now what is going on.

The film has a twist ending, a film technique created in *The Cabinet of Dr. Caligari*. However, before the audience reaches this, it can appreciate an example of the lack of communication in a couple during a crisis. The scene at the restaurant during their anniversary is the most illustrative. Malcolm and Anna had a good relationship, but the discovery that he could not help one of his patients makes their own relationship fall apart. Malcolm seems to be a perfectionist, something typical in people with traits of obsessive-compulsive personality disorder and not surprising in a child psychologist. His perfectionism helps him gain the city of Philadelphia's award but finding that he could not help one of his patients makes him surrender to a state of guilt that makes him dysfunctional even in his personal life. The only way he can restore his health is by helping another child in similar circumstances.

Cole is anxious, inadequate to his peers and isolated. He does not have a father and his mother is very busy. He is somehow neglected. His relationship with Malcolm becomes therapeutic. Malcolm helps him, listens to him and Cole is able to trust him enough to tell him his secret. Furthermore, Malcolm is able to help him by giving him advice on how to deal with his problem. After that, Cole becomes a happier child, and finds the courage to tell his mother about his supernatural abilities. Every time he sees dead people, the temperature in the room is lowered, something characteristic of demonic possessions.

When Malcolm finds out about Cole's secret, he wonders if Cole has childhood schizophrenia. While many children with anxiety can report seeing monsters, hearing things and talking to people, for the most part these reports are thought to be related to their anxieties and magical thinking rather than a psychotic illness. Childhood-onset schizophrenia is generally very rare and unless the child has genuine hallucinations – hears voices arguing, has structured hallucinations that she or he is able to describe in detail, coming from outside of the head – that are associated with other psychotic symptoms and a strong family history, an anxiety disorder should be suspected. However, the film concludes with an argument for supernatural abilities.

Malcolm and Cole help each other. The first has a need to help another child to relieve his own guilt and find peace. The second needs an adult who can help him find courage, and offer guidance and support. Malcolm represents a therapeutic father. Cole recommends Malcolm talk to Anna while she is dreaming. In grief it is very common to continue to have intrusive thoughts and dreams about loved ones.

Another example of more prolonged or pathological grief is the film *1408* (2007) directed by Mikael Håfström and based on the short story of the same name by Stephen King. In the film, Mike Enslin is a researcher and writer of the paranormal. After the death of his daughter, he separated from his wife and began researching the paranormal in an unconscious attempt to reconnect with her. However, Mike is an analytical person who does not believe in ghosts and is skeptical about what he researches. One day he receives an anonymous postcard from The Dolphin hotel in New York with the note, "Don't enter 1408." After being unable to book the room on the phone, Mike takes a flight to the Big Apple with the intention of spending a night there. The hotel manager, Gerald Olin, is unable to dissuade him from booking the room and Mike is finally able to access Room 1408. Soon after entering the room, Mike begins to experience visual and auditory hallucinations, which makes him believe he was given some psychedelic substance in the drink Olin had offered. Mike can see himself at the window in the building across the street, mimicking his gestures – an example of echopraxia, a prominent symptom of catatonia. He experiences several supernatural events and can see the ghosts of the people who died by suicide in that room through the decades and his own daughter. He manages to escape and save his life by setting the room on fire and is rescued by the firefighters.

In David Koepp's *Stir of Echoes* (1999), Tom is a charming man living in Chicago with his family who is hypnotized by his sister-in-law. The hypnotism session opens a gate to a different dimension. Now an intellectually disabled girl in the neighborhood named Samantha, who had disappeared six months earlier, can communicate with Tom in a rather hostile manner. Tom's son Jake also has special abilities to communicate with the dead. Samantha's evil actions won't stop until Tom discovers her body in the basement and solves the case of her murder. Once Samantha's perpetrators pay for what they did to her, the spirit will stop harassing Tom's family. In this film, the ghost of a person who was murdered is manifesting to the living to claim justice and revenge.

Many ghost films start from the basis of the existence of the soul beyond our physical form. As a result of injustice committed during the lifetime of the victim, the soul cannot appropriately rest in peace. This soul will be harassing a living human with a noble soul who can help them solve their problem before they can rest in peace and go to heaven. This theme is recurrent in a number of popular and horror films such as Guillermo del Toro's *The Devil's Backbone* (2001), Alejandro Amenábar's *The Others* (2001), Juan Antonio Bayona's *The Orphanage* (2007), James Wan's *Insidious* (2011) and Scott Derrickson's *Sinister* (2012).

The definition of the soul as the immortal essence of a being has been discussed since the beginning of civilization. In general, these films take a traditional or Catholic perspective of the soul, in which the dead remain conscious in soul form in the afterlife. This conception is much influenced by Plato's philosophy, which has been long considered the basis of the theses of Saint Augustine of Hippo – perhaps the most important theologian of early Christianity. In Book X of *The Republic*, Plato explains in a dialogue between Socrates and Glaucon (allegedly Plato's own brother) his take on the immortality of the soul. In the text, Socrates states that men who led a just life will receive their rewards after the mortal life is over. Glaucon is initially surprised that Socrates holds onto the immortality of the soul but Socrates elaborates on his arguments by stating that while illnesses attack the body and material things also become the prey of their own evil (rotting, rusting and so on) the soul is not destroyed by injustice (the soul's particular evil). Therefore the soul must be immortal. In the last section of the book Socrates argues that after death the souls of just men will be rewarded while the souls of unjust men will be punished. Socrates illustrates his theory via the myth of Er who, after death, was able to come back and share his journey of the afterlife. According to Er's story, the souls go to a place between heaven and earth where they are judged. While the just souls go to heaven to meet with the Fates, the unjust souls are punished to wander a thousand years beneath the earth. In fact the most unjust souls such as tyrants and murderers may remain beneath the ground for eternity.

A significant number of films about the paranormal take this approach to the soul as a somehow idealized form of the human in essence that continues to exist in a different realm after passing away. In that case, the spirits or souls of deceased people would retain full consciousness and memories of their earthly lives. They would also be able to interact with the living via the movement of objects, sounds, appearing as apparitions and so on. While most of the living would be apparently unaware of their existence and manifestations, children, animals and some people with special paranormal skills such as mediums would be able to acknowledge their presence, interact and communicate with them.

Amenábar's *The Others* employ a similar model of the soul. In the film Nicole Kidman interprets the character of Grace, a devout religious woman who lives with her two children in an English mansion at the end of World War II. Grace lost her husband in combat during the war and with the help of a few servants cares for her children Anne and Nicholas who have a disease that makes them photosensitive. Therefore there is no natural light in the house. Photosensitivity is generally rare and can have different etiologies. Today there are a number of drugs that can have photosensitivity as a side effect as with isotretinoin (a drug used in adolescents for the prevention of acne) and some antibiotics. There are some metabolic disorders such as porphyria, in which a protein called porphyrin – needed for the formation of hemoglobin – accumulates in the skin, causing sensitivity to sun exposure.

Anne and Nicholas begin to have contact with the ghost of a child named Victor. The house seems to be haunted by several intruders. The film concludes with a twist ending and brings up the issue of filicide (a parent killing their own child). Grace is found to have suffocated her children and shot herself. This is an example of filicide-suicide. According to an article written by internationally acclaimed forensic psychiatrist Susan Hatters Friedman for the *American Journal of Psychiatry*, up to 61 percent of children murdered under the age of five in the United States in the twentieth century were murdered by their own parents (30 percent by their mothers and 31 percent by their fathers). Women who commit filicide have been found to have a history of depression, psychosis, prior psychiatric service use, suicidal behaviors and substance abuse. These crimes tend to be more common in women from lower socioeconomic groups who are unmarried, give birth at a younger age or have had unwanted pregnancies. Filicide can take place in the context of gross negligence, recklessness or intentional acts. Filicide-suicide cases carry particular challenges since, for obvious reasons, it isn't possible to interview the mother and explore the nature of her homicidal behavior.

Insidious tells the fictional story of a child's struggles with Oedipus complex resolution and the impact that it has on his family. Dalton is a young boy who has moved to a new house with his parents Josh and Renai, his younger brother Foster and his newborn sister Cali. In one of the first scenes, Renai is holding Dalton while both look at old pictures in an album. Dalton tells his mom that she must be old, at least twenty-one. His mom smiles and caresses him. However, the mother–son sweet moment is interrupted by the newborn daughter Cali's cry. Renai leaves Dalton to attend Cali. In a different scene Dalton falls from the ladder and hits his head on the floor while exploring the attic. The next morning he is discovered in a catatonic state. His parents take him to the hospital, but no medical cause is found to explain Dalton's problem. The doctors allow them to take him home with the appropriate care. A few months later, Renai begins to see evil spirits in the house threatening Cali and begins to suspect that the house is haunted. She finally convinces Josh to move to another house. However, Renai begins to see ghosts in this new house even sooner than in their old house. Josh is hesitant to believe his wife but Josh's mother Lorraine – played by Barbara Hershey – tells him that she also feels the house is haunted. In the end they invite the medium and Lorraine's old friend Elise Reiner, who brings ghost hunters Specs and Tucker, to investigate the paranormal activity. Elise diagnoses the problem, explaining that Dalton's soul has traveled to a place located in a different dimension and now different spirits can use his body. Among these entities there is an evil demon trying to harm the family. Elise tells Josh that Dalton inherited the gift of traveling to other dimensions from him. In fact, she tells him that when Josh was an eight-year-old boy, Elise had to help him get rid of a female demon that haunted him. Elise will now induce a trance in Josh so that he can save his son. Once he finds his son, Josh will be able to fight his inner demons.

Insidious can be approached from the view of Freudian psychoanalysis as Dalton's story has interesting parallels with Freud's case of Little Hans. Dalton seems eroticized by the company of his mother as reflected in the first scene. Once his sister is born, Dalton is no longer Mom's priority as she has to focus her attention on Cali. Moreover, Dalton likely feels competitive tension with his father, as he fantasizes about becoming his mother's sexual mate. His catatonia seems to be of a conversive nature (conversive disorder refers to a neurological syndrome related to a psychological problem, something historically referred to as hysteria), but the doctors are unable to find a physical explanation for Dalton's problem. As in *The Testament of Dr. Mabuse*, Dalton is able to carry on his unconscious, previously repressed fantasies in his catatonic state. Out of resentment, he taunts his little sister and scares his mother through telepathic demonic manifestations. In a way, he is creating more distance between Josh and Renai; perhaps he unconsciously intends to cause a marital break-up and win the sexual competition. Similarly to Freud's interpretation of Little Hans, we could say that Dalton's neurotic catatonia might be the result of conflicts about his newborn little sister and sexual rivalry with his father, which can add a significant amount of castration anxiety. As with Little Hans's horse phobia, Dalton is able to come out of his catatonic state after he becomes closer to his father. At that moment all the evil spirits disappear.

Josh was traumatized as a young boy by an old woman. His memories, however, are repressed; he is not even consciously aware and is hesitant to believe the house is haunted despite Renai confronting him with clear evidence. During the trance to save his son, Josh reaches out to his unconscious inner conflict (symbolically represented as the demon of an old woman) and confronts it. Once he understands the root of the problem, there is a catharsis and Josh is restored to psychological wellbeing. Dalton seems to have a similar trauma that he inherited from his father. Recent scientific research on PTSD now shows that trauma can be inherited. Incidence studies show a higher risk of trauma in the children and grandchildren of traumatized persons. Emerging evidence suggests that DNA methylation, histone modifications, noncoding RNA regulation, and alternative splicing of mRNA provide an epigenetic means by which chronic stress and traumatic experiences alter gene expression to produce long-term changes in neuroanatomy, physiology and behavior. These epigenetic modifications caused by a stressful trauma can cause increased adrenal weight, heightened anxiety, exaggerated defensive response to threatening stimuli, memory impairment, increased arousal, and changes in cortisol related to dysregulation of the HPA axis. Although this is yet to be proven and understood, hypothetically, these epigenetic manifestations could alter parents' behavior and make an impact on the epigenetics of their own children. These modifications could hypothetically be present in the spermatozoids and eggs and passed genetically to their descendants. If this theory is proved right, Lamarckism, the ideas of French biologist Jean-Baptist Lamarck regarding the evolution of the species, will become possible once again and compatible with Darwinism, Charles Darwin's theory of the natural selection of species.

Japanese horror cinema leapt into the West in 1998 with *Ringu* (the Japanese term for ring), directed by Hideo Nakata. The film had several sequels and Western adaptations. It starts with the unexplained death of four teenagers. Rumor spreads that they died after watching a cursed videotape. Reiko, the aunt of one these teenagers, is a reporter who begins to investigate the case. She is intrigued with the nature of the teenagers' mysterious sudden death. In the video recordings of the retrieval of the dead bodies, their faces have a frozen expression of intense horror. One night Reiko goes to the hotel where the teenagers stayed a week before their death and discovers an unlabeled tape that gets her attention. She rents a cabin and plays the tape which shows a series of grainy black and white images including a woman combing her hair, a person covered with a sheet, a number of people crawling back and forth, and an eye with an inscription. After finishing the tape she immediately gets a phone call that states she has seven more days. Disturbed, she leaves the cabin and shows the tape to Ryuji, her ex-husband. Ryuji is a university professor and helps her with her research. They make a copy of the tape to analyze it in further detail and discover that the inscription is written in a dialect from the island of Izu Oshima. Reiko and Ryuji travel there and through a vision they discover that the tape was made by the vengeful spirit of Sadako Yamamura, the daughter of a psychic who lived there decades earlier and committed suicide after her supernatural powers were called into question. Sadako, who had stronger powers, was killed by her father. Reiko is able to find her body minutes before her seven days are up. As she survives, they believe the curse is over after they have found her body and resolved the enigma. However, the following day, Ryuji sees the ghost of Sadako crawling and leaving his TV to take a final look at him.

Ringu created a wave of interest in Japanese horror in the West. *Audition* (1999), *Pulse* (2001) and *Ju-on: The Grudge* (2002) are some examples of cult films that followed and influenced American films. In the American-made *It Follows* (2014), for example, similarly to *Ringu*, passing the curse onto someone else through sex is the only way to get rid of it. While *Ringu* leads the audience to believe that achieving justice will solve the curse, in contrast to traditional Western horror films, this turns out not to be the case. Reiko realizes that the only way to escape death is to make a copy of the tape and show it to someone else. Therefore while a logical explanation for Sadako taking revenge is shown to the audience, Reiko and Ryuji's discovery of the cause of the conflict provides no catharsis. Sadako will continue to kill for no logical reason, and passing the curse onto another random person will be the only thing that can save you.

Unlike Western horror ghost films, in which resolving the riddle causing the wrath of the vengeful spirit restores the harmony of the symbolic order, in *Ringu* the ghost's wrath will persist indefinitely even if the cause is found. In Asian horror films, very often a logical explanation is not provided. Often ghosts seem to appear and scare the living for no reason. They manifest and disappear without predictable pattern. This may be an artistic reflection of the historical differences between the East and the West in the way to approach and understand nature. According to Frank Perkins, a philosopher at DePaul University in Chicago, the West has taken an anthropomorphic theistic approach, seeing God and the spirits as images of themselves. According to Perkins, this may have led to the false belief that the human mind is uniquely suited to grasp the intelligible order of the world, which could explain the rise of science in Europe. In contrast, Perkins argues that while Asian territories had analogous views of anthropomorphic spirits, such views were breaking down at the time that philosophy began to appear in Asian countries. In that case, Chinese and other Asian thinkers had a much more humble view of humankind as merely one of the myriad things in nature. This approach, which for Perkins is more correct, would not provide enough confidence for humankind to generate the rise of science.

Australian film *The Babadook* (2014) by Jennifer Kent narrates the story of a special child, Samuel, and his mother Amelia. Samuel's dad had died in a car accident while taking Amelia to the hospital to deliver. Samuel has to live with the guilt of causing the death of a father he never met. He has behavior problems in school and has no friends. He is impulsive, hyperactive and due to his inattention commits reckless mistakes – the three domains of ADHD. Amelia seems overwhelmed by her role as provider and mother of a child with behavioral problems. One day, Samuel finds a book with the story of Mr. Babadook. By reading the story together, they invoke the monster that appears in the dark areas of the house. Babadook possesses Amelia to make her kill her son, but Samuel is a smart kid who knows how to handle the situation. Finally, the mother and son are able to keep the monster in the basement.

The Babadook depicts fear of the dark, one of the most common fears. The monster manifests only in dark areas, such as the closet, the corners or when the lights go off. Moreover *The Babadook* allegorically represents our own inner fears that we can't get rid of but must learn to control. In that sense, Amelia sends Babadook to the basement to keep him under control. Historically, in Christianity, our mundane temptations were attributed to the evil action of demons that we had to fight or control. Similarly, in acceptance and commitment therapy, the anxieties of the patient are referred as their monsters (like Babadook) that they must send to the back of the "bus" they are driving.

It Follows (2014) is a recent retro-like horror film directed by David Robert Mitchell. The film is a great example of persecution paranoia. Jay is an adolescent who has sex with Hugh after a few dates. After that Hugh sedates her with chloroform and ties her to a chair. When she wakes up he tells her that he just passed her a curse via sexual intercourse. Now it will be her duty to pass it onto someone else the same way in order to prevent being killed by a ghoul, which will be slowly but constantly coming after her in different human forms. Jay is initially confused about it but in her high school she sees an old lady following her, a lady who only she can see. That night at home, with her friends and sister, someone breaks the window and Jay sees a half-naked bleeding woman walking towards her. Jay locks herself up in her room but opens the door to her friends, who are followed by a scary tall man. After escaping a few times, she offers sex to the least scared of her friends, who is reckless, as he does not believe in the curse. As a result, one night he is killed by the ghoul of a middle-aged woman with dark hair and the curse is transferred back onto Jay. After a failed attempt to kill the thing by electrocution at the high school pool, Jay has sex with her childhood friend Paul, who has always had a crush on her. The film ends with the couple walking in the street of their suburb with a person following closely.

In *It Follows*, the same entity takes different forms to follow the person.

This is something described in psychiatric literature as Fregoli syndrome, usually in the context of psychotic or cognitive disorders. Persecution paranoia is the most common psychotic symptom. It consists of a person feeling that he or she is being followed or observed. At times, the person feels that someone is putting cameras in their house to watch them or that the police, FBI, CIA, the mob or other organizations are after them. Persecution paranoia is common in adolescents in the context of marijuana and or cocaine use. In general stopping the offending agent is enough for resolution of the symptoms, but in more severe cases antipsychotic medication may be needed. Often, this type of drug abuse can precipitate a first psychotic outbreak that evolves into schizophrenia.

The curse here is nevertheless transmitted via sexual intercourse. Anxiety about being infected with a sexually transmitted disease (STD) is usually more prominent in adolescents. In current society, the success of puritan thinking has increased the stigma of STDs and they have been used as a weapon against free sexuality. This may prevent embarrassed people from seeking help when needed. In people with obsessive-compulsive disorder and psychotic disorders, STD fear or paranoia is also common and can result in repeated visits to the physician's office even when results continue to come back negative. This kind of fear can often present as well in first-time cheaters. Their guilt acts out through somatic fears and risk of embarrassment via the transmission of an STD to their partner. Even when results come back negative, the person who has cheated may become obsessive about it and ritualistically go to different clinics to get tested. From a psychoanalytic point of view, this behavior could be interpreted as the partner's neurotic ambivalence and guilt at keeping the secret along with an unconscious effort to get caught and punished to relieve their guilty feelings.

CHAPTER 10

Slash Killers and Psychopaths

A PSYCHOPATH IS DEFINED as a person without morals, and who displays a lack of empathy, remorse and respect for societal rules along with extreme egocentrism. "Psychopathy," "sociopathy" and "antisocial personality disorder" are in general equivalent terms for the same condition. However, in clinical psychiatry, the term "antisocial personality disorder" is preferred. According to psychiatry's *Diagnostic and Statistical Manual of Mental Disorders* (DSM), the symptoms of this type of personality disorder include a pervasive pattern of disregard for and violation of the rights of others with at least three of the following behaviors: a failure to conform to social norms, deception as indicated by repeatedly lying or conning others, impulsivity, aggression, consistent irresponsibility and lack of remorse. The person must be at least eighteen years old but evidence of a history of these behaviors in childhood or adolescence is required for the diagnosis.

While a poor upbringing, history of physical and sexual abuse, and low socioeconomic status have been associated with risk of psychopathic behaviors, recent scientific discoveries suggest biological markers that may explain the personality disorder. In fact often individuals with antisocial personality have a family history of the same type of behaviors, hinting at a genetic cause. Recent neuroimaging studies comparing people with antisocial personality disorder and controlled groups have found thinning of the grey matter – neuronal loss – in several areas of the prefrontal lobe of the brain, in particular at the orbitofrontal cortex, an area that regulates planning and behavior control (an atrophy of this area would therefore result in impulsive behaviors). Individuals with antisocial personality often have a lack of fear response under stress and inhibited pleasure response. This is something that has made scholars hypothesize that people with antisocial personality disorder have abnormalities in communication between the prefrontal cortex and the amygdala (a subcortical area of the brain that modulates fear and emotion).

"Psychosis" and "psychopathology" are different terms and are not related to psychopathy, sociopathy or antisocial personality disorder. Psychosis refers to symptoms that interfere with reality testing such as delusions, hallucinations, and disorganized thinking (symptoms characteristic of schizophrenia and other psychotic disorders) and "psychopathology" is a term used to describe any symptom of the mind that may suggest a psychiatric disorder.

André de Toth's *House of Wax* (1953) was a remake of the 1933 Warner Bros.' *Mystery of the Wax Museum*. Due to the complexity of the plot and the psychology of its characters, the film is widely regarded as one of the early classics in the subgenre. Vincent Price stars as Professor Henry Jarrod, the official sculptor of New York City Wax Museum in 1890. Most of the wax sculptures depict important historical figures and moments such as Cleopatra and Mark Antony, the assassination of President Lincoln, Joan of Arc, Marie Antoinette and others. Jarrod is hesitant to succumb to his business partner Burke's request to make sculptures with more commercial themes such as horror or fantasy to lift their ailing income.

In one of the first scenes, Jarrod gives a tour to art patron Sidney Wallace who agrees to buy out the museum. That night, knowing that his business ambitions are over, Burke engages in a fight with Jarrod and sets the museum on fire, destroying all the wax figures and apparently killing him. Later, Burke tells his fiancée Cathy Gray that, after confirmation that Jarrod is dead, he expects a big payout from the insurance company which will allow them to go on a trip. However, after returning home, a disfigured man kills him and fakes a suicide by hanging. At that time it is revealed that Jarrod miraculously survived the fire and now works with two assistants in a new wax museum with a chamber of horror containing themes of historical and recent crimes to suit popular demand. Burke's fiancée Cathy is murdered and her body also mysteriously disappears from the morgue. One day Cathy's friend Sue arrives at the museum and is struck by the resemblance between Cathy and Joan of Arc. She suspects Jarrod and returns later to discover that the sculptures are modeled over the dead bodies of Burke and Cathy. Jarrod discovers her and tries to kill her and use her body for the wax model Marie Antoinette. In the altercation, Sue removes the wax from Jarrod, uncovering his true appearance.

Professor Henry Jarrod is initially portrayed as a well-mannered, educated man. He is passionate about his art of sculpting wax figures. As for many artists, Jarrod's wax figures are not only his major source of meaning in life but a way of coping with the existential anxiety of living in this world. In that way, art can help connect with the beauty of the world and, furthermore, contribute to it. Jarrod's art becomes the legacy that the artist leaves behind. In that case, his reaction after his partner Burke destroys his most precious creation is not surprising. Disfigured and without his collection, he plans a revenge proportional to the severity of his narcissistic injury. In *House of Wax*, an apparently harmless innocent artist is turned into a serial killer to satisfy his partner's ambitions. The artist's professional partner also becomes part of the project but not in the way the partner would have expected.

House of Wax also addresses the conflict between art and business. In the realms of a capitalistic society, when art becomes successful almost unavoidably it enters into conflict with the rules of the market. Often, artists can become stereotyped into specific themes, styles or subgenres. Once categorized under a specific subgenre, it can become a real challenge for artists to take on or develop unrelated projects. In this situation, artists may see themselves in a conflict between accommodating the market's demand and following their instinct and putting their success at risk. Jarrod, however, knows what he wants, and in view of the irreconcilable differences with his business partner, he seeks an art patron who believes in his ideas to buy him out. Burke is perhaps the real antisocial person in the film. He does not hesitate to try to kill his partner for money. In contrast, Jarrod is just fervently reacting in anger after seeing his dream destroyed by his business partner.

Though symptoms of antisocial personality can be quite common, only in rare cases does an individual commit murder. A person who commits three or more murders is often referred to as a serial killer. Perhaps the most popular historical case of a serial killer is that of Jack the Ripper. Also known as the "Whitechapel Murderer" at the time, he was believed to have killed up to eleven women – most of them prostitutes – in the impoverished area of Whitechapel in London between 1888 and 1891. The killer's method involved the slashing of their throats, abdomen and genitals and removal of internal organs. Though the murderer was never identified, there are some theories that suggest he was a person of high society who had good knowledge of anatomy and medicine. The case of Jack the Ripper has served as direct and indirect inspiration for multiple novels and films.

Another real case of a serial killer that has inspired many slash killer horror films is that of Ed Gein. The characters of Norman Bates from *Psycho*, Leatherface from *The Texas Chainsaw Massacre*, Frank Zitto from *Maniac* and Buffalo Bill from *The Silence of the Lambs* are at least loosely inspired by Gein's story. Gein grew up without friends, inadequate to his peers, and isolated. Gein's mother made him refrain from socializing as a child. His only friend and love in his life was his mother who died of stroke at the age of sixty-seven in 1945. Some years later Gein began exhuming the bodies of recently deceased women at the cemetery who resembled his mother to make masks and suits with their skins. This would magically allow him to "become his mother." Gein also killed two people but was found not guilty by reason of insanity and confined to a mental hospital.

In 1959, Robert Bloch wrote the novel *Psycho*, loosely based on the murders of Ed Gein. After his film *North by Northwest* (1959), Alfred Hitchcock became interested in directing what has been long considered the earliest example of a slasher film and one of his classics. Bernard Herrmann was commissioned for the famous soundtrack utilizing a string orchestra.

The story is centered on Marion Crane, a clerk in an office in Phoenix,

Arizona whose employer trusts her to deposit $40,000 in a bank. Marion instead steals the money and flies out to California with the intention of starting a new life with her lover Sam. During her trip she has to stay at Bates Motel for the night as she gets caught in a storm. The motel is decorated with stuffed birds and managed a by a peculiar man, Norman Bates, who lives with his mother Norma in a house next to the motel. With the construction of the highway the motel seems to have lost a lot of business and Marion so far seems to be the sole client for the night.

Norman offers her dinner and tells her about his mother who is mentally ill. Marion goes back to her room to take a shower and once there she is attacked by a female figure with a butcher's knife who slashes her fatally. Later, a private detective named Aborgast begins to investigate the crime and Marion's disappearance; his investigations lead him to Bates Motel. After interviewing Norman he asks to speak with his mother but he refuses to let him in. Aborgast enters the house without permission to talk to her and once upstairs he is killed by the same female figure. Subsequently, Norman tells his mother he has to leave her momentarily in the cellar until things calm down. Marion's sister Lila and Sam go interview the local sheriff who informs them that Bates' mother was killed with her lover ten years earlier. Concerned, they go to the house where Lila finds the preserved body of Norma Bates in the cellar, something that makes her scream hysterically. At that moment, Norman, dressed like his mother, appears in the cellar with a butcher's knife intending to kill her. However, Sam is able to stop him.

At the local courthouse a psychiatrist interviews Norman who has now assumed the personality of his mother. Norman, as Norma, declares against her own son fearing that she is going to be accused of all the crimes. The psychiatrist explains that Norman grew up with his mother who was his only social contact after the death of his father (this is similar to Ed Gein's story). After she found a lover, fueled by jealousy he committed a crime of passion and killed both his mother and her lover. In his mind this was unacceptable and, unable to cope with what had done, he tried to preserve his mother's body as if she was alive. As this was not enough to control his anxiety, he gradually became his mother. This new identity – Norma Bates – coexisted with his prior identity of Norman Bates but was not integrated in his mind. Whenever he found himself sexually attracted to a woman he would unconsciously become his mother to eliminate her. After being caught by the police, he became his mother to accuse her son and fall on the good side.

The iconic shower scene, in which Hitchcock decides to kill the main protagonist at minute 20, caused a wave of fear and shower hysteria for generations. The shower represents a very vulnerable moment in which a person is naked, defenseless, and now subject to the collective fear of being intrusively attacked by a person with a knife. The character of Norman Bates is a complex one. On one hand, his affliction has been classically pointed out as an example of double personality disorder, a type of dissociative disorder now known as dissociative identity disorder. In this case, the person with dissociative identity disorder has two behaviors that are usually contradictory and not integrated in their consciousness. For instance, Norman seems unaware that he, instead of his mother, has committed the crimes and vice versa.

Psychoanalytically, this can be approached from the domains of the object relations theory developed by Melanie Klein. According to this school of thought, the objects are the caregivers or, at an earlier stage of development, the parts of the caregivers (such as the breast, the hands and so on) that influence the baby's emotions towards development of a psychic structure. For Klein newborns go through two main developmental stages: the schizoid-paranoid position and the depressive position. During the schizoid-paranoid position that lasts approximately from birth to six months the baby is unable to integrate the good with the bad and as a result will be splitting good and bad and will be consequently paranoid and fearful of the potential "bad part objects" (for example, a bad breast with bitter milk). Later, the baby will gradually be able to integrate the good with the bad and therefore will learn that Mom has good and bad things and that she is neither perfect nor evil. This stage is called the depressive position (the term refers to the discovery that his or her mother is not all good and has some bad aspects). Nevertheless a good resolution of this stage will lead to the ability to integrate the good with the bad in the world. When a good resolution of the depressive position is not reached a defense mechanism called "splitting" can emerge. In splitting, a person cannot integrate the good with the bad and constantly switches from idealization to devaluation of people. Splitting is certainly common in personality disorders, especially in borderline personality disorder, a condition that has been highly associated with dissociative identity disorder.

Whether Norma Bates was a good mother or not, we will never know but what seems to be more evident is that Norman's introjection of his own mother is an example of the introjection of a bad object. When he talks with her, she is abusive, dismissive, demanding and mentally disturbed. Perhaps Norman's feelings of abandonment after she found a lover resulted in a furious narcissistic rage that led to the passionate crimes. After that, a bad introjection of her served to make him feel less guilty about what he did. Norman also has voyeuristic fantasies – a repeated theme in Hitchcock films – and observes the young woman in the bathroom through a hole in the wall. These erotic fantasies represent the libidinal drives towards his own mother, which raises the inner tension and the intrapsychic conflict. The elimination of the new libidinal object via murder under the identity of the bad object, his mother, will be the easiest way for him to cope with the conflict. In addition to voyeurism, Norman has transvestic fantasies that strengthen his new identity as his mother.

Norman's mental pathology seems very severe. In the film there are no portrayals of the splitting behaviors characteristic of personality disorder. He instead is portrayed as a shy, socially inept person. He lives alone, has no friends and seems to have had social fears and anxiety since early childhood. He is rather concrete and has a constricted and bizarre affect. He seems to hear the voice of his dead mother and develops the delusion that he can become his own mother. He preserves a dead body in his house, believing that it is his mother, alive, and in the end, he believes he has become his mother. All these symptoms fit better in a picture of schizophrenia. In that case, Norman's inability to cope with so much intrapsychic conflict would surrender him into a psychotic state.

Psycho marked the path to a new trend of a psychopathic and slasher killer film genre. In 1974, Tobe Hopper directed the low-budget film *The Texas Chainsaw Massacre* which, though banned in a number of countries, soon became a cult classic. To date three sequels, a remake and two prequels, have followed. Similarly to *The Exorcist*, at the start a message states that the film is based on a true story to create a sense of realism and increase the horror feeling. Congruent with the 60s and 70s hippie style, Sally, her disabled brother Franklin and three more friends, Jerry, Kirk and Pam, travel in a van to investigate the apparently ritualistic vandalism of their grandfather's grave. While on the road they pick up an unpleasant hitchhiker who takes a Polaroid picture of them and demands money for it. After they refuse to pay he grabs Franklin's knife and slashes his arm. Prior to that he had cut himself with the same knife just for the sake of it. After they force the hitchhiker out of the van they arrive at their grandparents' old house. The neighbors, however, are cannibalistic. One of them – Leatherface – hits Kirk in the head with a mallet when he enters the house to ask for gas. Pam also enters the house and finds a room full of bones. Leatherface catches her and hangs her on a meat hook where she watches as he cuts Kirk into pieces with a chainsaw. Next, Leatherface kills Jerry who has gone to the house in search of his lost friends. As Sally and Franklin are calling for their friends, Leatherface appears from the dark, inserting the chainsaw into Franklin's abdomen. Sally manages to escape to a gas station but the owner turns out to be part of the neighbor's family. He ties her up and takes her to the house. There she sees the hitchhiker again and Leatherface, who is now dressed as a woman. The body of the grandmother is preserved upstairs – a reference to Norma Bates – and the grandfather, who is barely still alive, is fed with fresh blood. Finally Sally is able to leap from a window and run to the nearby road. Leatherface is unable to catch her and waves the chainsaw with frustration as she watches him from the back of the pickup truck that rescued her.

In the film, the first aspect of interest from a psychiatric point of view is Franklin's frustration with his own disability. Though not clearly stated, it appears that he was not born disabled. As the others go to the pool and do things he is unable to do, he declines. Whether the accident that occurred to him was remote or recent, he is still having a hard time coping with his inability to walk.

The hitchhiker picked up in the van raises the theme of self-mutilation without a suicidal intention, a behavior that is thought to release inner anxiety and tension. This type of deliberate self-harm is more common in the context of poverty and lack of education – as in the film – and also in teenagers or people with borderline personality disorder, who lack the more mature or adaptive coping skills to deal with stress.

The character of Leatherface, loosely inspired by Ed Gein, used skin from dead people to make himself a mask. He lacks vocabulary and the ability to communicate and seems intellectually disabled. Though his face is always covered – something that makes the character even more terrifying – in one scene we can see a thin upper lip with delayed development of his teeth and enamel; this, together with his other intellectual features, would suggest fetal alcohol syndrome, a condition that is also more common in the context of isolation, poverty and lack of education. He practices transvestism as he serves dinner. In the house there are no women, as his grandmother is dead and his mom is not in the picture. Similarly to Norman Bates, Leatherface introjects and assimilates his mother by dressing like her.

Kirk is hit in the head with a mallet and immediately begins to have a seizure. This is a common manifestation of traumatic brain injury, and is likely the cause of his death. From a cultural point of view this family's cannibalistic practices would not necessarily allow them to meet the criteria for a psychiatric diagnosis. Though they seem to have some sense of wrongdoing – they take steps to avoid getting caught and the father is unable to kill – the practice of cannibalism for survival could be accepted in their very isolated environment. This idea has been recently revisited in Jim Mickle's cannibal film *We Are What We Are* (2013).

Following the success of *Psycho* and *The Texas Chainsaw Massacre* and influenced by giallo cinema, there was a demand for more releases of this new slasher film horror genre. *Halloween* (1978) by John Carpenter became one of the first American slasher films in which an unknown killer slashes a group of adolescents one by one with a bladed object. A film with this storyline, influenced by giallo cinema, usually concludes that the current events are linked to something wrong that happened in the past and generally leaves only one survivor – usually a female virgin. Carpenter's film is set on Halloween night in 1963. That night, a six-year-old Michael Myers stabs his teenage sister after she has sex with her boyfriend. Due to this he is locked up in a sanitarium under the strict supervision of psychiatrist Dr. Sam Loomis but manages to escape at the age of twenty-one.

Michael goes to his old town of Haddonfield, Illinois and begins stalking his sister Laurie who was adopted by the Strode family. In the meantime Dr. Loomis also travels to the town fearing that Michael will kill on Halloween night. Michael steals the gravestone of his mother and begins killing each one of Laurie's friends. In the end he makes every effort to kill his sister, who does not know she is Michael's relative, but Dr. Loomis – the psychiatrist – saves her.

Michael Myers shares some elements with Norman Bates. Both use a butcher's knife to kill their victims, and stab them in a similar manner. Both have voyeuristic fantasies. Michael observes his victims long before he takes action. Like Leatherface, Michael covers his face with a mask – a reference to the boogeyman – and does not talk. As a kid and as an adult, Michael stabs his victims after they have sex. In giallo cinema this is the general fate of the sinner, whereas from a psychoanalytic perspective, Michael's behavior can be understood as a need for penetrating the victim because of an inability to engage in sex or as an impulse to remove the object that triggers unacceptable behaviors.

Following the DSM criteria, Michael Myers is portrayed as an individual with impaired social skills and communication. He is unable to talk. He lacks theory of mind and empathy. His pattern of interests seems limited to finding his sister and killing whomever he finds. In this case an argument that Michael Myers suffers from autistic disorder could be made.

Halloween is one of the first films to portray a hero psychiatrist, Dr. Sam Loomis. He saves the girl, the virgin, at the very last moment and shoots the assassin. He goes beyond his duty and responsibility to stop the evil.

While Norman Bates, Leatherface and Michael Myers are loosely inspired by the real story of Ed Gein, perhaps the fictional character that is more closely related to the real person is Frank Zito from the film *Maniac* (1980) by William Lustig. In the film, Zito suffered abuse in his childhood from his mother and in adult life. Now he hires prostitutes in order to kill them. He later keeps their scalps as his trophies (perhaps in an attempt to prevent his mother from abandoning him one more time). Unlike the others, Zito's character is more realistic and believable, something that enhances the feeling of terror. Other examples of films that portray a more realistic serial killer are *Henry: Portrait of a Serial Killer* (1986), *American Psycho* (2000) and *Wolf Creek* (2005).

After the commercial success of *Halloween*, Sean S. Cunningham had an idea for a new slasher film, a type of film that according to the director would "make you jump out of your seat." Victor Miller was commissioned for the script and Harry Manfredini for the musical score. The film's title was going to be *A Long Night in Camp Blood* but Cunningham finally chose the name *Friday the 13th* (1980) after rushing an advertisement into *Variety* magazine. The movie was filmed in the towns of Blairstown and Hope and the still active No-Be-Bo-Sco summer camp in New Jersey.

The story takes place during the summer at the camp at Crystal Lake in 1958. One night, while a group of teenagers is singing religious songs, a couple sneaks to a barn to have sex but are followed by an assailant, who kills them. Twenty years later, Annie is trying to reach the camp but she is warned by a madman, some locals and a driver about the curse of the camp and the drowning of a boy, Jason Voorhees, a year before the murders of 1958. Annie ignores the warnings and she is soon slashed in the neck by an unseen killer before reaching the camp (as in *Psycho*, the main character dies early in the film). In a different scene, a group of teenagers meet at the camp by the lake. Those who engage in sex die first but the killer eliminates everyone but the final virgin.

Cunningham used the same point-of-view technique as Spielberg's *Jaws* to shoot the killing scenes. The assassin is not discovered till the end and turns out to be Pam Voorhees, the mother of Jason Voorhees, the kid who was bullied and drowned in 1957, avenging the death of her son. In the sequels, Jason comes back to life as an adult. He hides his facial deformities with a bag – another reference to the boogeyman – and later with a hockey mask and kills all the teenage visitors with a machete. As in *Psycho*, the story is based on a complex mother–son relationship; the father is not in the picture. After his mom dies, Jason preserves her head in a hut and believes she could be alive, as shown in the first sequel. However, in this case, mother and son love and care for each other. To an extent, *Friday the 13th* is a mother–son love story.

Pam Voorhees exacts revenge for her son's death on his anniversary. In American culture, anniversaries are especially significant moments of revival of grief. Jason's facial features (shown in the end of the first and third films of the franchise) and lack of cognitive skills are consistent with an intellectual disability, likely due to some kind of congenital metabolic disease. Children with physical and intellectual disabilities are at high risk for becoming victims of bullies. Jason was bullied and ended up drowned at the lake in front of all the other kids.

Before making *Friday the 13th*, Sean Cunningham had produced Wes Craven's directorial debut *The Last House on the Left* (1972). Soon, Craven's works, including titles such as *The Hills Have Eyes* (1977) and *Swamp Thing* (1982), were acclaimed, but his biggest success would arrive with his popular supernatural slasher horror film *A Nightmare on Elm Street* (1984). In the film, Nancy Thompson, her boyfriend Glen Lantz and her friends and couple Tina Gray and Rod Lane are having nightmares about a burnt man who has a glove with razor blades. The situation becomes alarming when the nightmares go beyond dreams and Tina Gray is violently killed by the man known as Freddy Krueger who also kills Rod and Glen as they sleep. Nancy battles her fate by not falling asleep but as days pass by, it becomes harder and harder to stay awake. At some point, her mom reveals that this man they dream about was actually a child murderer in the neighborhood. After he was caught and released by the judge due to lack of evidence, the parents decided to take justice into their own hands and burnt him alive.

In *A Nightmare on Elm Street*, the four protagonists are isolated and

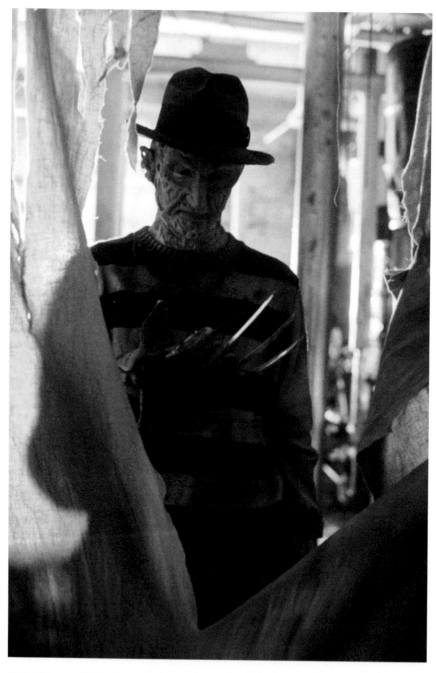

FIGURE 10.1 Burnt Killer Freddy Krueger Manifests in the Dreams of the Traumatized Adolescent of Elm Street (*A Nightmare on Elm Street*) Licensed by Warner Bros. Entertainment Inc.

neglected by their parents. For instance, Nancy's mother is distant and shallow and has a boyfriend who does not give her attention either. Her father is a strict and cold police officer who gets angry often. Tina's father has died and her mother is in Vegas with a boyfriend. Glen's mother is away and when he calls her, he has an audio recording set up to stop the conversations at his will. Clinically, their nightmares could be explained in the context of PTSD. Freddy Krueger was a child murderer; he probably killed some of the protagonist's brothers when they were young or not even born. Perhaps they had even been attacked by Freddy when they were children. PTSD is characterized by recurrence of the traumatic memories in the form of intrusive thoughts. These thoughts are unpleasant and anxiogenic and recur in the form of flashbacks or nightmares. As in our film, these dreams can be very vivid. Even when the traumatic memories are repressed, the thoughts may appear in the form of unpleasant dreams that the individual cannot always understand. Other times, trauma can cause symptoms of derealization. In these scenarios, the individual can feel detached from reality and confused about what is real or not. All these symptoms are depicted in the characters of *A Nightmare on Elm Street*. Nancy is able to overcome Freddy Krueger by convincing herself that he is not real and accepting that he is just a dream, the result of her imagination. However, consistent with the post-Cold War paranoid horror, the film concludes with Freddy's return.

Influenced by giallo and other slasher films, the issue of sinful teenage sex is also brought up. Tina dies right after having sex with her boyfriend who becomes the next victim. Nancy has a crucifix in her room that protects her and stops Freddy's evil actions. To preserve virginity gives you the best chance of survival.

Freddy was a serial killer. He committed the most horrible crime: killing children. In a remake (2010) Freddy is portrayed as a pedophile. After being killed for his deeds he comes back for revenge. Freddy kills for fun and has no empathy for his victims. Despite the atrocities he has committed, he can appear as superficially charming. All these features are characteristic of antisocial personality disorder.

In the original film, Freddy's story is introduced to Nancy by her mom. Freddy was a child killer in the neighborhood who, after being discovered and captured by the law, escaped legal prosecution because the police had illegally entered his home. This injustice angers all the parents in the area who hunt him down and set him on fire, burning him alive. However, his spirit survives in the dreams of the teenagers of Elm Street. In *Dream Warriors* (1987), which was written by Wes Craven, although he left the project after seeing how many of his ideas were being cut out, we discover more biographical information about Freddy. Here Freddy's background is revealed by the mysterious nun who repeatedly appears to the psychiatrist, Dr. Gordon. This nun turns out to be Amanda Krueger, Freddy's mother, who was a nurse at the asylum which featured in the film. At the time the asylum housed the most dangerous criminally insane. One night, Amanda was accidentally locked up in the asylum for a weekend and repeatedly raped by all the criminals; she miraculously survived but became pregnant. The result was Freddy Krueger.

The character of Freddy Krueger was conceptualized by Wes Craven, inspired by an old creepy man he saw once in his childhood in the street through the window and by a bully in his school named Freddy. In this case, two traumatic experiences of the director's childhood sublimate into one of the most influential characters in the history of horror cinema. In the documentary *Never Sleep Again* (2010), Craven states that at that time he had also read an article in the *Los Angeles Times* about a refugee boy from Cambodia who refused to fall asleep due to having disturbing nightmares – likely due to traumatic experiences in Cambodia – and tried to stay awake for days at a time. When he finally fell asleep, the parents felt the crisis was over, but the boy woke them up in the middle of the night screaming. The parents later found him dead in his bed.

Another film that has interesting social implications is *Freddy's Revenge* (1985), the first sequel to the original motion picture. Though it was not the intention of the filmmakers, this film has been pointed out by critics as having a clear subliminal homoerotic message. In fact actor Mark Patton stated he probably would have been the first male scream queen of horror.

In the fourth film of the saga, *The Dream Master* (1988), a dog – interestingly named Jason – is able to resurrect Freddy with his urine. The idea of bodily fluids such as urine having magical properties is related to traditional folkloric beliefs shared by different cultures. In this case, Jason's urine magically channels Freddy's spirit back into the world of the living. The fifth film, *The Dream Child* (1989), reflects on the anxieties a woman can go through during pregnancy.

Today nightmares in people with PTSD can also be treated with behavioral psychotherapy. For example, in the realms of cognitive behavioral therapy it is understood that after a traumatic event a person can have negative thoughts – cognitive distortions – around the circumstances surrounding the events, like patients blaming themselves for things they could not have really changed. In that case, a therapist will try to help the patient replace these negative thoughts with less distressing ones. The therapist will challenge how accurate or realistic the patient's negative thoughts are in order to replace them with more positive thoughts.

Cognitive behavioral therapy is not only a valid therapy for PTSD, it is the most widely used evidence-based therapy for the treatment of anxiety and depressive disorders. According to Aaron Beck, the founder of cognitive behavioral therapy, the root of people's depressive and anxiety-related symptoms originates with these negative thoughts, which he called cognitive distortions. Some examples of cognitive distortions are black and white thinking (if things don't go perfectly there is a sense of total failure), overgeneralization (if something bad happens, we expect it will happen over and over again), catastrophizing (exaggerating the importance of insignificant events), mind reading (a person feels that others always have a negative perception about them), fortune telling (anticipating a negative outcome) and many others. In cognitive behavioral therapy, the counselor will challenge the cognitive distortions with the use a technique called Socratic questioning. Similarly to the way Socrates used to challenge people in Plato's dialogues, the therapist will challenge the accuracy of the patient's negative thoughts. Through cognitive exercises and homework exercises, the patient will gradually learn how to reframe these thoughts in a more positive and adaptive manner, and ultimately he or she will see how the anxiety or depressive symptoms related to their negative perceptions are alleviated and become more tolerable. In PTSD, the decrease of intensity in anxiety symptoms related to the trauma will also decrease the intensity and frequency of nightmares.

Another popular therapy for the treatment of PTSD is eye movement desensitization and reprocessing (EMDR). In this therapy, while talking about the traumatic events, the person will focus on other activities such as eye movements, hand taps or sounds. The therapist may move his or her hand and the patient will follow the movement with the eyes. Ultimately, the patient will learn how to dissociate himself or herself from the traumatic experiences and therefore the traumatic symptoms such as hypervigilance, avoidance, recurrence or nightmares will decrease.

In more severe cases of PTSD, the clinician may use medication as an adjuvant to psychotherapy with the idea of maximizing recovery, in that case selective serotonin reuptake inhibitors (SSRIs) and other antidepressants can be helpful. Also, in the specific treatment of nightmares, a medication called prazosin has been shown empirically helpful. This drug blocks the adrenaline released in the body via blocking of the alpha receptors. In addition to helping alleviate anxiety and subsequently nightmares in patients with PTSD, this blockage of alpha receptors helps decrease blood pressure in patients with hypertension and the size of the prostate in patients with benign prostate hypertrophy. More recently, a drug called D-cycloserine, which was initially synthesized as an antibiotic for use against tuberculosis, has been found helpful in extinguishing fear in patients with PTSD and other anxiety disorders as well as enhancing learning in patients who receive exposure therapy for anxiety disorders. In this therapy the person imagines the hypothetical situation that causes anxiety and processes it with the assistance of the therapist.

Some people grow up in circumstances of repeated and continuous physical and/or sexual abuse and gross neglect. As a result, they have great difficulty establishing good quality relationships with family, friends or at work, something that can be very disabling and affect the ability to function in society. These patients are thought to have a complex form of PTSD. Severe and prolonged trauma has been related to dissociative symptoms (amnesia, depersonalization or derealization) and, in extreme cases, dissociative identity disorder. In this last disorder, the person will dissociate the trauma to the point of unconsciously creating a different self, unaware of the traumatic events. In repeated trauma in childhood, the person can face significant challenges to develop a mature personality ready to face the stressors of daily life. This may involve difficulties using adaptive defenses and instead splitting (seeing everything as either all good or all bad), projection (unwanted feelings are displaced onto another person) and projective identification (unconsciously projecting the bad feeling onto the other person, so that the other person behaves negatively) will become the major defenses. In these cases, the person may lack self-identity, will have unstable relationships and due to their inability to face responsibilities may suffer chronic thoughts of suicide and expose themselves to dangerous situations. These are core symptoms of what we call in psychiatry a borderline personality disorder. In these severe cases, other more complex therapeutic modalities such as mentalization-based treatment, psychodynamic therapy or dialectic behavioral therapy may be more appropriate. Obviously, trauma can cause disabling symptoms that interfere with a person's ability to function in society. Nonetheless, overcoming trauma in life can certainly help a person become resilient and more prepared to face other adversities. The stories of very successful people are often determined by a need to overcome very difficult challenges and traumatic events in life. Still scholars don't agree on which factors for a person facing adversity are determinant as to whether he or she will become resilient and stronger or dysfunctional and depressed.

In Wes Craven's horror classic, the nightmare is the central element of horror. Often during a nightmare a person has no control over the fear, and only after waking up can they regain a sense of control. A nightmare by definition is a frightening or unpleasant dream. The meaning of dreams, whether they are good or bad dreams, has been a subject of debate since the beginnings of psychoanalysis. Today, it is well known that all animals sleep, even the most primitive ones such as jellyfish, and most mammals have dreams, despite lacking the language to narrate the content of their dreams. One of the first persons to analyze and approach the content of dreams was Sigmund Freud, who in 1900 published *Die Traumdeutung* (The Interpretation of Dreams). According to Freud, while dreaming, the preconscious was more relaxed and allowed for unacceptable thoughts of the unconscious mind to become conscious. Freud defined dreams as "the royal road to the unconscious." In this case, dreams were the result of "wish fulfillment" of the unconscious desires that are repressed by the superego. During psychoanalytic sessions, the patient and the analyst could discuss the symbolic meaning of the images they consciously remembered during the day. For Freud, however, dreams were often presented in a "transformed" rather than clear and straightforward fashion. The meaning of this transformation was to hide unwanted thoughts from our awareness so that we or other people wouldn't know about these unacceptable thoughts or desires. As a result, what Freud called the "manifest dream" (the content of the dream that we consciously remembered) was distorted and the therapist needed to analyze it through free association in order to interpret and understand the real dream or, as he defined it, the "latent content" of the dream. For example, in his famous case, The Wolfman, Freud concluded that this dream was probably related to his patient having seen his parents having sex doggy style at an early age. This interpretation relieved Pankejeff's anxieties, and for Freud was a resolution of the patient's neurosis. Today in modern psychodynamic psychotherapy, dreams are also considered important. However, in contrast to Sigmund Freud's methodology, modern therapists agree that the manifest dream should be considered the main source of information rather than attempting to access the latent content through free association. For most of us, dreams have a meaning that concerns our own subjective psychological lives. Very often we dream about either our desires or our fears. Sometimes our dreams have a straightforward interpretation, other times the manifest content of our dreams can be more symbolic or difficult to understand. In these cases, the assistance of the therapist can certainly be helpful.

Another film that deals with sleep problems is M. Night Shyamalan's *The Visit* (2015). Here, in contrast to many other slasher movies, an elderly and apparently inoffensive couple becomes the serial killer psychopaths. *The Visit* is filmed as found footage. In the movie, Paula is the mother of Becca and Tyler and sends her children to a farm to meet their grandparents. Paula had abandoned the house fifteen years earlier after falling in love with a man of whom her parents did not approve. However, she reassures the children that their grandparents are very nice people and they are going to spend a memorable week with them. Once at the house, the children begin to notice eccentric behavior; Pop Pop, their grandpa, spends too much time in a barn and has bowel incontinence. Nana, their grandma, often scares them when she plays with them, puts her shirt upside down, and at times appears confused, with catatonic stares. She does strange things such as asking Becca to get all the way into the oven to clean it. Moreover, the children notice she sleepwalks at night, crawling, running or scratching the walls. One night Tyler leaves the camera outside to discover there's something really wrong with their grandparents.

Initially grandpa Pop Pop explains to Tyler and Becca that their grandma suffers from a sleep disorder associated with old age. Several behaviors described in *The Visit* are related to psychiatric disorders of the elderly. Advanced age is the single most important factor associated with the increased prevalence of sleep disorders. Sleep-related phenomena reported more frequently by older than by younger adults are sleeping problems, daytime sleepiness, and daytime napping. Clinically, older patients have higher rates of sleep apnea or other breathing-related disorders. Nana seems to have a sleepwalking disorder, which usually happens a few hours after falling asleep and is characterized by walking in the sleep and inappropriate behaviors such urinating in the closet, sleeptalking and screaming if combined with sleep terrors, violent attacks and no recall of the event on the day after.

In the midst of the production of multiple slasher films, Tom Holland directed *Child's Play* in 1988. In this case, the killer is Chucky, also known as the Lakeshore Strangler in Chicago. After being shot by a police officer, he is able to transfer his soul by practicing a voodoo ritual on a "Good Guy" doll right before dying. Soon, he will start seeking revenge while looking for a new host before turning into a doll with human qualities. Chucky lacks empathy or remorse, is egocentric, and attempts to manipulate everyone – even an innocent kid. Chucky portrays a clear case of antisocial personality disorder.

In 1990 Rob Reiner directed *Misery* based on Stephen King's novel (1987) of the same name. According to the narrative, Misery is the central character of a series of successful romantic novels written by Paul Sheldon. After finishing his last novel in the small town of Silver Creek, Colorado, Sheldon is caught in a blizzard while driving back to New York City and suffers a car accident. Annie, a fan who was following him, rescues him, takes him home and takes care of him. She claims to be his number one fan. Grateful for her saving him, Paul allows Annie to read his most recent novel. Annie, however, is disgusted by the obscene vocabulary used by Sheldon in the novel and can't help but have an outburst while she is feeding him. After that she buys Sheldon's last novel of the *Misery* saga, *Misery's Child*, in the town store. Annie initially praises the book but one night she wakes Paul up in the middle of the night in anger due to discovering that the character of Misery dies at the end of the novel. In that moment of anger she reveals that she lied to him when she told him that she has been in contact with her agent and the authorities. No one knows where he is; Paul has actually been kidnapped. Annie locks the door and does not allow him to leave the room. She buys paper and a typewriter, suggesting he starts writing a new novel, *Misery's Return*. Paul agrees and in an attempt to control her unpredictable behaviors, he tells her that he will dedicate the novel to her as a reward for saving his life. Annie seems to buy Paul's story and gets excited with the idea. During one of Annie's journeys to town, Paul is able to sneak out of the room by using a hairpin in the lock and discovers a scrapbook of newspaper clippings in which he finds that Annie was fired from her job as a nurse after being suspected of a number of infant deaths. Paul then realizes his life is in danger. When Annie comes back, she drugs Paul and once he wakes up she tells him that she knows he has been out of his room and breaks his feet with a sledgehammer and a board to prevent him from doing it again.

After the local sheriff, who begins to suspect Annie based on her past behaviors, discovers Paul in the house, Annie kills him and proposes she and Paul both commit suicide. She knows that more police officers will come. Annie begins to believe Paul loves her too. In order to gain some time, Paul suggests finishing *Misery's Return* before committing suicide. After finishing the novel, Paul asks for a glass of champagne and a cigarette as part of his usual ritual every time he finishes a novel. Annie knows this and provides him with his requests but before she can read the final chapter, Paul burns the book and hits her on the head. They fight but he is able to kill her with the typewriter. Eighteen months later, Paul meets with his agent in New York. Paul is now a more successful mature writer but still has flashbacks and hypervigilance symptoms from his trauma in Colorado.

Paul becomes a better writer after his traumatic experience. Trauma can sometimes make someone depressed or dysfunctional but, on other occasions, if the person is able to overcome obstacles and learn from experience, trauma can make someone more capable of new challenges. This is called resilience and it has gained the attention of psychiatrists, in particular child psychiatrists, during the last few years. Psychiatrists try to find elements within patients who face adversity to promote resilience.

Annie has an obvious problem with controlling her impulses. Her temperamental outbursts are consistent with an intermittent explosive disorder, a disorder characterized by recurrent outbursts with inability to control impulses including verbal or physical aggression with or without destruction of property. As portrayed in the film by Annie, the outbursts are out of proportion to the psychosocial stressors that cause them. Annie feels unable to regulate her mood when frustrated. She ends up breaking Paul's feet and puts his life at risk on several occasions. Kathy Bates, the actress who portrays Annie, won an Academy Award for Best Actress for her brilliant performance.

Intermittent explosive disorder is a type of impulse control disorder, like pathological gambling (impulsive play), kleptomania (impulsive stealing), trichotillomania (impulsive hair picking) and pyromania (impulsive setting of fires). In all of them, the individual affected suffers from an inner tension that builds up until the impulse can no longer be controlled. The inner tension is only relieved after the impulse becomes manifest. Despite not being classified under impulse control disorders, other impulsive behaviors such binge drinking, binge eating and purging in eating disorders or sexual paraphilia (in which a person's sexual arousal and gratification depend on fantasizing about and engaging in sexual behavior that is atypical and extreme) are considered by scholars as impulse control disorders.

Biologically in intermittent explosive disorder and other impulse control disorders that carry aggression there is thought to be abnormalities in the orbitofrontal cortex and the amygdala. Studies of the CSF of aggressive impulsive individuals have shown a decrease of 5-HIAA, a metabolite of the neurotransmitter serotonin. Therefore, this finding has set the basis to support the use of selective serotonin reuptake inhibitors (SSRIs), a class of antidepressants, which increase serotonin levels in the brain by inhibiting its reuptake for metabolism in the neurons, in the treatment of intermittent explosive and other impulse control disorders. However, other drugs such as mood stabilizers and antipsychotics have been tried with success too. Despite psychotropic agents being much used in clinical practice, to date the gold standard treatment for impulse control disorders is cognitive behavioral therapy. In this therapy, the patient meets with the therapist regularly to learn and practice more adaptive and mature ways of coping with frustration.

In addition to intermittent explosive disorder, Annie seems to have clear symptoms of erotomania or de Clérambault's syndrome. More common in women than in men, erotomania is the delusional belief that a person is loved by someone, usually of a higher rank or social status, despite no evidence. The syndrome was first described by French physician Gaëtan Gatian de Clérambault in his 1921 review *Les Psychoses Passionelles*. De Clérambault was a physician, psychiatrist, painter, photographer and writer. He was also awarded the Croix de Guerre after serving in World War I and unfortunately took his own life with a firearm.

Erotomania generally has been classified under primary erotomania, which would be consistent with a delusional disorder or secondary to another mental or medical illness. Traditional literature supports the use of an old typical antipsychotic called pimozide. However, the use of this drug is mainly based on single case reports. While there is little research on erotomania, risk factors include social isolation and few sexual experiences. The two seem to be evident in the character of Annie. Occasionally this syndrome has been associated with stalking behaviors, something that could lead the patient to committal in a forensic institution. Annie has a long-standing obsession with Paul Sheldon and his romantic novel series. She identifies herself as his number one fan. Nonetheless she initially does not believe that Paul is in love with her. Gradually through the film, she begins to develop ambivalent feelings about it. At times she wants to believe it, other times she realizes that she is too naïve and that it is not possible as she is not an attractive woman. However, at the end of the film her overvalued ideas seem to reach a delusional level. She believes she and Paul love each other, and she has to kill the local sheriff to prevent him from taking her lover. She understands that suicide (in a Romeo and Juliet fashion) is the only way they can stay together for eternity.

Another atypical case of a killer is portrayed by child actor Patty McCormack as an eight-year-old child named Rhoda in *The Bad Seed* (1956). It has been long recognized that genetics contribute to antisocial behaviors, and in general it is assumed that the earlier these behaviors appear the stronger the genetic component of the personality disorder. Though biologically antisocial personality disorder cannot be accounted for by a single factor, studies comparing monozygotic and dizygotic twin brothers suggest a strong genetic factor. Even if a child with a strong genetic component for antisocial behaviors was adopted by a family providing an optimal environment, the behaviors could still appear. This deterministic biological model for antisocial personality was already anticipated in *The Bad Seed*. The film is based on William March's novel of the same name. At the beginning of the film, Colonel Kenneth has to go to Washington DC, leaving his wife Christine with their adoptive daughter Rhoda. The girl is superficially loving but demanding and manipulative. At school, Claude, one of Rhoda's classmates, drowns in the lake during a school picnic. The case is not resolved, but Rhoda has no emotion about the tragedy. It is also known that Claude had been the winner of the penmanship medal, a trophy that Rhoda believed she deserved. Christine begins to suspect her daughter, especially after finding that Rhoda is the biological daughter of a famous serial killer. Feeling that there is no hope for her daughter, as she has inherited the bad seed, she will try to end her life before she grows old and the crimes escalate. The film's theme is also related to *The Omen* (1976) and *Damien: Omen II* (1978) in which Damien is also an adopted child who shows antisocial behaviors very early on. In contrast *We Need to Talk about Kevin* (2011) portrays a family in which there is no evidence of antisocial behaviors yet one of the children begins to show these behaviors. The film does not provide a rational explanation for Kevin's psychopathic behaviors. Once Kevin becomes an adolescent he commits a school massacre after killing his family, an event that was not anticipated by anyone. Though more rare, at times individuals with antisocial personality disorder do not have a family history of antisocial behaviors and have had good parenting. David Slade's *Hard Candy* (2005) portrays a fourteen-year-old girl who meets an adult online who fantasizes about teenagers. Once they meet, she sedates him, ties him up and attempts to castrate him to punish him for his potential criminal behaviors. In *Hard Candy*, castration anxiety becomes a real thing.

The first horror film to win the Best Picture Academy Award was *The Silence of the Lambs* (1991) by Jonathan Demme. The film is based on the novel by Thomas Harris (1988) of the same name. In contrast with *Halloween*'s benevolent Dr. Loomis, the psychiatrist here is Hannibal Lecter, a cannibalistic serial killer.

The movie's protagonist is Clarice Starling, a young FBI agent in charge of interviewing Hannibal Lecter at the Baltimore State Hospital for the criminally insane. Clarice is assigned this work to see if she can get Lecter to cooperate in the search for Buffalo Bill, a Midwestern serial killer who has just kidnapped the daughter of a US senator. Lecter agrees to cooperate in exchange for Clarice satisfying his curiosity about her childhood and personal life. In the meantime, the FBI finds the bodies of more people who seem to have been killed by the same person they are looking for. Dr. Frederick Chilton, the psychiatrist at the State Hospital, secretly records the conversations between Clarice and Hannibal Lecter. After discovering that they are attempting to offer him a fake deal in order to get more information, Chilton talks to the senator on his own and offers Lecter a real deal in an attempt to get the credit for finding Buffalo Bill.

The characters in the film are very complex. In the first place, Clarice Starling is a lonely person. From the conversations with Hannibal Lecter we infer that her mother died at an early age. After that, her father, a police officer, became the world to her but was shot by two burglars. However, he survived for a month before passing away. Clarice has flashbacks about her dad's funeral when going to the funeral of one of the victims. She reveals to Lecter that once she became an orphan, she was adopted by an uncle to live in Montana on a ranch but she ran away one night after she was awoken by the sound of lambs being slaughtered. She says that she tried to release them but they were disoriented. Then she took one of them and ran away a few miles until she was caught by the local sheriff. Her uncle would not allow her to return home after that and she was raised in an orphanage. In the first interview, Lecter figures out that she went into the FBI in an attempt to escape from a miserable life. Clarice is an attractive young woman and is conflicted about being perceived as a sexual object. Dr. Chilton, for instance, is one of the first people to make an inappropriate comment on that. Lecter also wonders if her superior, Jack Crawford, is attracted to her and wonders about the feelings she has for him too.

Dr. Chilton is narcissistic. He is probably jealous that Hannibal Lecter is smarter than him and so treats him very poorly. Chilton uses disproportionate punishment against Lecter and eavesdrops on his conversations with the intention of unjustly getting recognition by the media.

Buffalo Bill has some commonalities with the Ed Gein type of serial killer. He skins his victims to make himself a female dress. He is transsexual and was rejected from several clinics in which he tried to change his sex. Lecter had met him with his partner years before he began killing. According to Lecter, Buffalo Bill was not born antisocial and his behavior is the result of systematic rejection at all levels. Bill is a victim of repeated trauma and has an unstable self-image. For him the moth symbolizes his own transformation. As inferred from Lecter he had unstable relationships, impulsivity, anger and emotional instability. These features are characteristic of borderline personality disorder, a disorder that in part is thought to be caused by repeated trauma since childhood. Nonetheless, Buffalo Bill ends up killing people and shows little of empathy for the victims, something that suggests that he also has traits of antisocial personality disorder.

Hannibal Lecter is a psychiatrist and a cannibal. He does not respect the norms, and kills people to eat them. He also shows no empathy for his victims. He has an antisocial personality with sadistic features. He is very intelligent, highly educated and very fond of art history, Italian architecture of the Renaissance and classical music. In a memorable scene, he cites Marcus Aurelius's *Meditations* when guiding agent Starling: "What is it in itself? What is its nature?" Hannibal Lecter can be polite, attractive and charming but he is also very manipulative. According to Dr. Chilton his heart rate did not change much after eating the jaw of a nurse. Lack of vegetative response (e.g. increased heart rhythm) in situations that would cause excitement is a major feature of antisocial personality disorder. As a result, the person with antisocial personality may need to carry out behaviors in search of the same excitement and pleasure that a normal person would need, such as cannibalism, extreme violence, and the like. Lecter, however, likes Clarice. He has a psychological voyeuristic attraction towards her and wants to learn as many details as possible about her personal life. He intentionally touches her when he gives her a file at the end of the film – while still in the cage – knowing that it may be the last time they see each other. He wants to help her find Buffalo Bill but he also wants to help her psychologically. Hannibal Lecter carries out therapy with Clarice without her being aware of it. He has a psychodynamic approach and wants to understand her childhood trauma, hidden under the scream of the lambs at night. The lambs in fact are a symbolic representation of her father who died after a month of agony accompanied by a helpless girl – Clarice – who could not do anything to save him. Clarice became an FBI agent so as to sublimate her frustration about her childhood, her youth and the circumstances surrounding her dad's death.

After the success of *The Silence of the Lambs*, the popularity of the classic slasher film franchises began to decline. However, Wes Craven brought this type of film back to the mainstream with *Scream* (1996), a new concept of slasher film combining horror and humor. In *Scream*, the protagonists are aware of the rules in the slasher horror film genre (don't have sex; don't drink; and don't say "I'll be right back"). The film satirizes all slasher horror movies while introducing a new idea to the genre – the killers now are real people and have an emotional connection with their victims. This new concept makes *Scream* even more horrific.

In *Scream*, a year after the murder of Sidney Prescott's mother, an anonymous killer who wears a ghost mask kills two high school lovers. After this, the killer begins stalking Sidney and continues to kill other people in the peaceful town of Woodsboro, California. The main suspect is her own boyfriend but he is released due to lack of evidence. Sidney begins to understand that these murders are in some way connected to the murder of her own mother. As she is grieving her mother's death she begins to accept the fact that her mother was not the way she would have liked her to have been; she was promiscuous and cheated on her father. At some point Sidney reveals to her boyfriend that she fears becoming like her mother, something that has been preventing her from losing her virginity. In *Scream*, we can see how Sidney gradually accepts grief and trauma at the time that she understands the psychological causes of her inability to develop intimacy. Sidney's case is an example of psychological healing, resilience and adaptive coping with trauma.

As portrayed in Craven's films, trauma can result in recurrence via intrusive thoughts and nightmares. In a situation where trauma is very severe or impairing, the person may not be able to deal with it and so dissociate. In this case, the traumatized person detaches the trauma from reality and from the self. While, clinically, dissociative amnesia is the most common type of dissociative disorder, in film, dissociative identity disorder – also known as double or multiple personality disorder – is the most frequent one. During the 90s, dissociative personality became a hot topic in the scientific and popular domains. As a result a number of films came out, contributing to this topic. *Primal Fear* (1996) and *Fight Club* (1999) are examples of it. In the horror genre, *Identity* (2003) by James Mangold tells the story of ten strangers who seek refuge in an isolated motel during a nasty rainstorm – a reference to the Bates Motel. The strangers are mysteriously killed one by one, something that induces a paranoid fear among them. In a twist ending, a psychiatrist discovers via old videotape recordings that these people are the different identities of a serial killer.

Hostel (2005) and *The Purge* (2013) take the concept introduced by Wes Craven in *Scream* – a regular person being the killer – to a higher level. In *Hostel* the killers are very wealthy people who have a regular life. Having every pleasure this world can offer within their reach, they want to push the limit even further. They pay to go to Slovakia to enjoy the experience of torturing and killing a regular tourist. In *The Purge*, the government designates a twenty-four-hour interval in which killing is permitted. The goal is to get rid of the homeless and poor people who won't be able to defend themselves, somehow purging society. Here, anyone can potentially become a killer.

American Psycho is an American-Canadian cult movie directed by Canadian Mary Harron in 2000. It is based on the novel (1991) by Bret Easton Ellis with the same name. Only a year after the release of the novel, film producer Edward Pressman got the rights to the novel and attempted to recruit David Cronenberg to direct the film but he turned down the project. After that Harron as director and Christian Bale as lead actor were commissioned. However, at that time Bale was less known to the audience and Pressman made a final attempt to replace Harron with Oliver Stone and Bale with Leonardo DiCaprio. In the end DiCaprio abandoned the project to work with Danny Boyle on *The Beach* and Pressman ended up hiring Harron and Bale.

The film is set in Manhattan in the 1980s, a time in which the economy of the United States was undergoing significant economic changes under the administration of US President Ronald Reagan. These changes, also referred as Reaganomics, attempted to decrease government expenses, reduce federal taxes and reduce inflation. Reagan proposed a model of free market economics with less regulation. These changes carried a temporary increase in GDP growth and employment and a decrease in poverty. Nonetheless the total public debt doubled.

The sector that had most benefit from Reaganomics was Wall Street which saw an explosive growth in the stock market. After 1982, the stock market would begin an ascent that would not really come to an end until 2000. Nonetheless, today, different scholars and critics see this unsustainable growth with increased debt and lack of regulations, which allowed subprime lending by banks, as the main reason for the worldwide financial crisis of 2008.

During the 1980s, a number of young professionals with a college education moved to Wall Street to work at the stock market and became very wealthy. This group, referred to as yuppies, were educated, well paid, self-absorbed and enjoyed fancy clothes and restaurants and the expensive cultural options offered by the large city.

In *American Psycho*, Patrick Bateman is a wealthy investment banker – a yuppie – living in New York. Like his colleagues, he is narcissistic and driven by vanity. His relationships are superficial. They compete for having the nicest business card which for them is a big deal.

Bateman is very jealous of one of his colleagues, Paul Allen, who is more stylish, has a nicer business card and confuses him with another person. As a result of his narcissistic injury, Bateman kills Allen one night at his apartment. Through the movie, Bateman becomes increasingly concerned with his appearance and his status in the group and begins to lose contact with reality. One night he invites two prostitutes and after having sex with them (while looking at himself in the mirror all the time), he physically abuses them. On a different day he invites a college friend and manages to convince one of the same prostitutes to come back to the apartment, offering more money. He ends up killing his friend and the prostitute by throwing a chainsaw at her when she is running away down the stairs. Bateman gradually loses touch with reality, he is distracted at work and all he does is to draw images of rape, murder and mutilation. At this point, we understand he is having a severe mental breakdown. One night, after killing a few people in the street and at the building where he works, he realizes that his life has fallen apart and there might be no return. In a cathartic attempt to relieve his anxieties he will attempt to confess but society might not be ready for that.

American Psycho portrays a superficial society without values. People are driven by an egoistic self-directed pleasure principle which seems to be the result of the materialistic society resulting from capitalism. Like his colleagues, Bateman has character traits of narcissistic and antisocial personality disorder. Nonetheless, we see how he gradually loses contact with reality and has a major breakdown. In the film we never find out if his murders are real or just delusional fantasies. Bateman seems to have a pathological grandiosity, feeling on the top of the world, an increased energy, an expansive affect, hypersexual behaviors, goes on spending sprees, and feels a decreased need to eat and sleep and at times an extreme irritability that takes him to aggression and murder. Though there is no clear timeline in the film, these symptoms seem to last for at least a week or two until he has a questionable restoration to health at the end. This cluster of symptoms would be consistent with a manic episode, something that would be enough to make a diagnosis of bipolar disorder. While during a manic episode there is a higher tendency to abuse alcohol or drugs (cocaine and alcohol are present through the film), people from the upper and upper-middle classes are thought to be at increased risk of bipolar disorder.

Historically, "mania" was a term used in ancient texts to describe a furious state with uncontrolled rage and strength. However, today mania describes a specific cluster of symptoms in the context of a mood disorder. While it is believed that most people with manic episodes have had or will have at some point in their lives episodes of depression, the latter would not be needed to meet criteria for bipolar disorder.

According to the DSM, in order to meet criteria for a manic episode, a person must have a distinct period of abnormally and persistently elevated, expansive, or irritable mood, lasting at least one week (or any duration if hospitalization is necessary). During this period of mood disturbance, the person must have at least three or more specific symptoms that need to be present to significant degree during the entire episode. These symptoms can be inflated self-esteem or grandiosity; a decreased need for sleep (for example, feeling rested with only three hours of sleep); being more talkative than usual or feeling the pressure to keep talking, having a flight of ideas (stating many different things or ideas with pressured speech that do not seem connected) or having a subjective experience that one's thoughts are racing; distractibility (for example, attention is too easily drawn to unimportant or irrelevant stimuli); an increase in goal-directed activity (either socially, at work or school or sexually) or psychomotor agitation and excessive involvement in pleasurable activities that have a high potential for painful consequences (such as engaging in unrestrained buying sprees, sexual indiscretions, or foolish business investments). In order to meet full criteria, the person must have significant impairment in occupational functioning, social activities or relationships with others or must need hospitalization, and the symptoms must not be explained by the use of drugs or other substances or a direct physiological cause (like thyroid disease). A manic episode often happens concomitant with psychotic symptoms (such as delusions or hallucinations) that can be congruent or incongruent with the person's mood.

Historically, mania and depression were seen as two different entities, but in the late nineteenth century, German psychiatrist Karl Kahlbaum used the term "cyclothymia" to refer to stages of mania and depression as the same illness and, a little later, Emil Kraepelin compiled all the knowledge from the

French and the German schools of psychiatry to describe what he termed "manic-depressive illness" or "psychosis." Kraepelin's description of the phenomenology and course of the disease is still the one used by psychiatrists to diagnose bipolar disorder.

Today, it is widely regarded that the pathophysiology of bipolar disorder is strongly biologically driven. Research in neuroscience shows that people afflicted with bipolar disorder have several dysfunctional changes in their neurotransmitters (dopamine, serotonin, norepinephrine, GABA and glutamate), sleep patterns, inflammatory biomarkers and the HPA. More recently, conceptual and experimental evidence suggests that abnormalities in the regulation of signal transduction cascades and neuroplasticity could more primarily underlie the pathophysiology of bipolar disorder. In addition, data obtained from neuroimaging studies have shown frontal and subcortical changes compatible with other severe mental illnesses such as schizophrenia or psychotic depression.

In clinical practice and popular culture there has been significant confusion about bipolar disorder. A number of people with borderline and narcissistic personality disorders have been wrongly diagnosed as suffering bipolar disorder. This may have been influenced by the media too. In the last few years, a number of celebrities and artists with a substance abuse problem, narcissistic maladaptive defenses and relationship problems have reported to the media that they are suffering bipolar disorder. While it is certainly possible to have concomitant bipolar disorder and a personality disorder (the case of Patrick Bateman could well represent an example of it), bipolar disorder is thought to be less prevalent. In general, most people with personality disorder don't meet the DSM criteria for bipolar disorder.

Another factor that may have contributed to the confusion is the negative connotations that a diagnosis of personality disorder can carry, such as a sense of guilt and responsibility for the diagnosed person's actions and consequences. In contrast, a diagnosis of bipolar disorder, which is perceived as a more biological illness, has gained more acceptance by people with personality disorders. This diagnosis could potentially excuse the person from the responsibility of his or her actions. In that sense, this "social demand" from the elite and upper classes for being diagnosed with bipolar disorder may have contributed to the diagnosis overlap. Another determining factor that has contributed to the confusion has been the drug-centered paradigm of care. Over the last two decades, many psychiatrists have abandoned psychotherapy to focus on more profitable, less time-consuming medication management and left appointments for psychotherapy to other providers. Insurance companies reimburse more for the number of visits than for the time spent with the patient. Since there is no clear psychopharmacological indication for personality disorders or mere behavioral disturbances, the system has favored an increase in the rate of mood disorder diagnoses, including bipolar disorder. Many psychiatrists and patients are not satisfied with the current model of care and demand a swift return to a more balanced biopsychosocial model of psychiatric care. In the United States, recent changes in Current Procedural Terminology (CPT) coding and evidence of the benefits of psychopharmacological and psychotherapy care by a sole provider provide hope for a better model.

In the field of psychiatry, there has also been a lot of debate by scholars as to whether people with personality disorders, who tend to have emotional dysregulation, anger outbursts and risky behaviors, have some subclinical form of bipolar disorder. In fact, while psychotherapy is considered the gold standard treatment in personality disorders, the psychopharmacological treatment of both disorders does not differ much as both end up getting treated with mood stabilizers such as anticonvulsants and antipsychotics. Furthermore, the drug lamotrigine – an anticonvulsant mood stabilizer – has been found to be quite helpful in the treatment of both bipolar disorder and mood lability in people with personality disorders.

One of the most sophisticated characters of all the serial killers is John Kramer, the jigsaw killer from the *Saw* franchise (2004–2010). Kramer is a man of morals and lives according to his principles. He is intelligent, perfectionistic and highly qualified. After being diagnosed with terminal cancer, he becomes angry and feels betrayed. As a result, he challenges the Creator and decides to make justice on his own.

According to the stages of death and dying elaborated by Elisabeth Kübler-Ross, anger comes after denial in patients diagnosed with terminal illness. Kramer externalizes his anger onto others and begins to kidnap people who according to his own beliefs are immoral or don't respect social norms. They are people who have chosen irregular ways of life and do whatever they want. For this he designs very sophisticated machines and through the jocular puppet Billy, he gives them a choice. They can save their lives but have to make a big sacrifice first (such as killing another person in violent way, or deforming their own body). One of his first victims in the first film is Dr. Lawrence, his surgeon. He meets Kramer's victim profile. Dr. Lawrence is narcissistic, egocentric, charming and seems to have little empathy for the suffering of his patients and his family. He wants to cheat on his wife and is a distant father. Probably, Kramer's guilt is relieved by giving his victims an option of saving themselves. His perfectionism, inflexibility and detailed sophisticated killing machines are suggestive of obsessive-compulsive personality disorder.

James Wan's *Saw* seems related to David Fincher's *Seven* (1995). In both, a perfectionistic killer has the grandiose idea of making some kind of moral justice through a detailed and macabre plan. *Seven* is set in a dreadful oppressive atmosphere. William Somerset is the detective lieutenant in the homicide section of the police department in a crowded, polluted city. He is partnered with young detective David Mills who recently moved to the city with his wife

Tracy. They are commissioned to investigate two atypical murders, one of an obese man who was forced to eat until his stomach exploded and the other of a rich attorney who died of fatal blood loss. They realize the two murders might have been caused by the same person and follow clues that take them to the apartment of the possible third victim. At the apartment they find an emaciated body on a bed that despite having a mummified appearance turns out to be miraculously alive. Somerset and Mills realize that these three crimes have in common the fact they are cardinal sins (gluttony, avarice and sloth). From the public library they get the name of a man named John Doe who has been borrowing books about the seven deadly sins and find him at his apartment, but he is able to escape. The detectives are too late to prevent the death of the "lust" victim, a prostitute raped with a razor blade and the "pride" victim, a supermodel who after being disfigured is given the choice to call 911 or commit suicide with pills. Finally, Doe gives himself up but blackmails them by saying he will plead insanity unless the three of them drive to a specific place. Mills, who is more passionate, convinces Somerset to do what Doe asks (he does not want him to plead insanity) and they arrive at a place in the middle of the desert where there is a box containing the head of Mills' wife. At that moment, Doe confesses his envy of Mills hoping that he will become "wrath" and kill him.

In the Catholic Church, a sin is defined as a morally bad act. In his "Summa Theologica," Saint Thomas Aquinas lists the seven deadly sins that must by all means be avoided: gluttony, avarice (greed), sloth, luxury, vainglory (pride), envy and wrath. According to the important theologian and philosopher these vices have an exceedingly desirable end so that in his desire for them, a man goes on to commit many sins, all of which are said to originate in those vices which are their chief source. In that case, it is not then the gravity of the vices in themselves that makes them deadly but rather the fact that they give rise to many other sins. Ever since Saint Thomas Aquinas, these seven deadly sins have not been changed by theologians and Church leaders.

Catholicism accepts the ontological argument that all humans have free will; therefore, sins are voluntary acts by definition. Sins in general were divided into original, mortal and venial. The original sin – disobeying God's commands by eating an apple from the tree of wisdom in the Garden of Eden – was committed by the voluntary act of Adam in the Book of Genesis in the Bible. In contrast, venial and mortal sins are considered personal and voluntary. Whereas venial sins are lesser sins that can impede our connection with God, a mortal sin can carry a total separation from God, a spiritual death of the soul. Mortal sins must have knowledge, free will, and concern a grave matter. For Catholics, humans have the ability to reason and have free will. In that case, for a deliberate sin there must be full knowledge on the part of the intellect and full consent on the part of the will in a grave matter. In contrast, an involuntary transgression of the law even in a grave matter is not a formal but a material sin. The *Catholic Encyclopedia* comments on the possibility of committing a philosophical sin, which is a morally bad act that violates the natural order of reason, but does not alter the divine law. Instead, a theological sin is a transgression of the eternal law. For example, people with atheistic tendencies who either deny the existence of God or maintain that He exercises no providence in regard to human acts.

In this Catholic definition of sin, free will is a necessary construct. In that case, those deprived of reason such as people with severe mental illness would potentially be considered innocent of their committed sins, as they would lack the ability to discern between good and evil. However, in the field of neuroscience, many scholars now state that free will is incompatible with the physicalist model of the mind. For neuroscientists, the human mind is the result of a combination of multiple biological factors vulnerable to environmental influences. In this construct, a person would not be able to be held responsible for their actions, as their behavior would be technically biased by many variables such as genes, hormones, physiological states, diet, weather and so on. These factors are for the most part considered unconscious to the person, or at least beyond their control. Therefore, a person could not theoretically be held fully responsible for their actions. A person who believes in the Catholic conception of sin and in the physical and deterministic model of behavior embraced by neuroscience would technically live in contradiction unless he or she dissociated faith from science.

From an ethical point of view, our ability to punish people who commit crimes or who violate rules would be tested too, unless that punishment is ethically supported by the potential benefit that the majority of the community would potentially get from it. Punishment (such as putting criminals in jail and so on) would therefore be made not for the benefit of the person (who technically lacks free will and would therefore become another victim) but for the benefit of the potential third parties affected by the person's deviant behavior.

In psychiatry, the theses of philosopher Immanuel Kant are used to sustain the ethics of the psychiatrist's ability to remove a patient's autonomy. For Kant, people are born with an innate capacity for morals, and presumably have the ability to reason to decide between rightful and wrongful behavior. In Kant's arguments, reason is necessary to support the ability to have autonomy. In the case of a person who has a mental illness that interferes with their ability to reason at an acceptable level, the person's autonomy could ethically be removed. In clinical practice, psychiatrists often find themselves in the dichotomy of whether or not to remove a patient's autonomy for the benefit of themselves or others. For example, those with severe psychotic symptoms such as paranoia or hallucinations whose symptoms would put them at risk of hurting a third party, or put themselves in a situation in which they could be victimized by others, or those who due to a severe depression may wish to die or kill themselves, may be hospitalized against their own will until with the appropriate care their judgment is restored.

The current popular physicalist and deterministic model of human behavior proposed by many modern neuroscientists is incompatible with the concepts of autonomy and free will. In this case, not even decision-making would be a valid construct in psychiatry. Killers and criminals could not theoretically be held responsible for their actions. Instead, their biological structure, together with their adverse experiences in their lives impacting their epigenetics, are to be blamed for their misdeeds. Nonetheless, an existentialist approach to the issue of freedom may take the question to a different level. According to existential philosophy, the existence would precede the essence. Therefore, whether, based on recent advances in neuroscience, humans have free will or not would not be the important question. The real issue would be what we, as human beings, want to decide in regards to the definition of human freedom. In this case, each human would have to make the ultimate decision whether or not to embrace the existence of human free will. This decision would carry a tremendous responsibility and a subsequent existential anxiety, since the direction taken would not only define the person at the individual level but each decision would contribute to what all of humankind does in regards to the question of human freedom.

CHAPTER 11

Zombies

THE WORD "ZOMBIE" OR "zonbi" originates from the Kongo word *nzambi* which means "soul." The transformation of people into zombies is a superstitious ritual practice in the "voodoo" or "vodou" religion and a ritual practice in Haiti, Louisiana and other places with French colonial heritage.

For a long period, Haiti lacked the infrastructure to be truly governable from Port-au-Prince, its capital city. At that time, the countryside was in effect governed by voodoo secret societies that controlled the rituals of zombification. According to Haitian tradition zombies were lifeless beings resulting from the effects of a nerve toxin administered by members of a secret society. This was presumably done clandestinely to destroy overly offensive members of the community. Later another rumor spread that these clandestine groups could open the grave of a "dead" person, resuscitate them, and banish them from the area. Sometimes brain damage would result from either the toxin or the lack of oxygen during entombment.

The zombie character was central to Haitian folklore. According to Haitian people, a dead person could be turned into a zombie with the use of magic powers. A zombie would preserve similar functions to other living humans such as eating or sleeping but would have a diminished level of consciousness, apathy and abulia. Once turned into a zombie, the person could be used as a slave. In Haiti, zombies are not aware of their status as zombies unless they are fed with salt. In that case, all of a sudden, the zombies will understand their new status and run away immediately to the place where they came from. In order to prevent a body from being turned into a zombie, the dead body has to be buried upside down with tape over its mouth.

Swiss anthropologist Alfred Métraux (1902–1963) spent several weeks in Haiti and alerted locals to his interest in searching for a real zombie. In his book *Voodoo in Haiti*, he relates his experience one day when in the middle of the night several people woke him up to show him what they believed was a real zombie that was wandering around. After careful observation, Métraux concluded that that person was not a zombie but an individual with severe intellectual disability. In the 1980s, Harvard ethnobotanist Wade Davis traveled to Haiti in the search of the psychoactive drug that could turn people into zombies. In his book *The Serpent and the Rainbow* (later made into a motion film by Wes Craven in 1988), he presents the case of Clairvius Narcisse, a man who had been a zombie for two years as a result, according to Davis, of the use of a substance called tetrodotoxin, a neurotoxin derived from puffer fish and other fish, as well as the plant datura, which produced a powerful hallucinogen, and cultural beliefs.

Haitian zombies or slave zombies had a significant impact on cinema. In 1932, the Halperin brothers directed *White Zombie*, an independent film based on a book by William Seabrook that narrates the story of a young woman who is gradually turned into a zombie under the influence of a malevolent voodoo master (played by Bela Lugosi). A sequel and several other films with voodoo zombies followed in the next decade. Some examples are *The Ghost Breakers* (1940), *King of the Zombies* (1941) and *I Walked with a Zombie* (1943).

The conception of the modern zombie as a recently dead flesh-eating person came with the release of George Romero's masterpiece *Night of the Living Dead* (1968). Romero cited *Carnival of Souls* (1962), *Repulsion* (1965) and *The Last Man on Earth* (1964) as the major influences for his film. *Carnival of Souls* was directed by Herk Harvey. It was an independent horror film in which a young lady experiences the harassment of a ghoul (played by the director himself) after surviving a terrible car accident. A psychiatric interpretation of the movie could be that the woman developed PTSD after a car accident. *The Last Man on Earth* was an adaptation of Robert Matheson's novel *I Am Legend*. The book narrates the story of Robert Neville, a person who is apparently the sole survivor of a major pandemic that has turned the population into vampire-zombies. Neville is depressed and abuses alcohol to cope with isolation. He works in his lab with the goal of finding a cure. Two other film adaptations of the novel that came in the following decades are *The Omega Man* (1971) and *I Am Legend* (2007).

The script for *Night of the Living Dead* was the result of collaboration between George Romero and his friend John Russo. In fact Russo had the idea that undead would be hungry for flesh. The main character, Ben, was played by African American actor Duane Jones. This was a novelty at the time and an important step considering that the film was made at the end of the era of the Civil Rights Movement. Since the word "zombie" was still associated with the voodoo zombie, Romero and Russo used the word "ghoul" for their creatures.

The film starts at the cemetery of Evans City, Pennsylvania. The siblings Barbara and Johnny visit from the city to put flowers on their father's grave. When Johnny starts taunting Barbara ("They're coming to get you Barbara"), both see a strange man in the horizon who attacks Barbara as she is returning to the car. Johnny tries to help his sister but he falls, hitting his head against a headstone. Later on, the ghoul chases Barbara who can't start the car but is

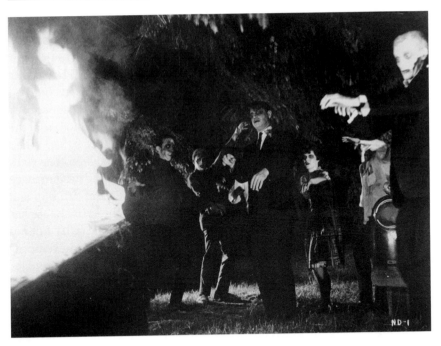

FIGURE 11.1 A Group of Living Dead Are about to Eat Some Flesh (*Night of the Living Dead*)

able to escape by removing the car's handbrake. Then she arrives at an aban-doned farm, where she encounters some stuffed animals in the living room – a reference to *Psycho* – and other similar people wandering outside the house. Upstairs, she finds a dead rotting body. She tries to leave the house when Ben arrives and protects her from other wandering ghouls who attempt to enter. After that, Barbara falls into a catatonic stupor and becomes unre-sponsive, something certainly possible under excessive emotional distress. Ben seals the doors and windows. The radio warns about these wandering subjects and advises everyone to stay home. At some point, Ben finds that in the cellar there are more people: the Cooper family – Harry, Helen and their daughter Karen, who is ill after being bitten by one of the creatures, together with a teenage couple, Tom and Judy.

Soon, the tension arises between the occupants as they try to figure out the best plan to survive. Harry tries to convince them that everyone should hide in the cellar but Ben is hesitant and sends him downstairs, stating that he is the boss upstairs. Ben finds a TV and when he turns it on, they learn that the deceased are coming back to life and eating the flesh of living people. It is postulated that this phenomenon is happening as the result of radioactive contamination. Once they hear that there are some places that offer refuge and medical care, Ben makes a plan to escape in a truck but Tom accidentally spills gasoline on the vehicle, setting it on fire and killing both Tom and Judy. Right after, the flesh eaters start to feed on their bodies. Harry locks the door and does not allow Ben to re-enter the house. Once he gets in, Harry takes the rifle and threatens Ben. An altercation between the two begins but Ben is able to take the rifle again and shoots Harry. An injured Harry goes back to the cellar to find that his daughter has just died and turned into one of the creatures. After collapsing, the daughter begins to feed on her father. When Helen goes to the cellar, she is shocked by the scene. Her daughter then stabs her with a trowel, killing her. In the midst of all this, the living dead manage to enter the house; one of them is Johnny who takes Barbara with him and she is subsequently devoured by the dead. By this time, the entire house has been invaded by the ghouls and Ben has to lock himself in the cellar, but not before killing Karen and Harry who are now living dead too. The next morning Ben hears the gunshots of the sheriff and his deputies killing the zombies and goes to them, excited that he was able to survive. However, he is mistakenly identified as a living dead and killed.

The *Night of the Living Dead* introduced the modern concept of the zombie as a flesh eater and the possibility of turning a person into a zombie through bites. The cause of the plague is considered radiation activity, an idea that links the film to the post-atomic bomb and Cold War paranoia film genre. After all, the Cold War was still going on at the time the movie was made. The film has been considered among the most scary of all time. Dead people coming back to life hungry for flesh, a child eating her parents, a brother turning into living dead to kill his sister and the tragic ending were very horrific but innovative scenes. The film was conceptualized with two more sequels, *Dawn of the Dead* (1978) and *Day of the Dead* (1985).

Dawn of the Dead was the biggest commercial success of the trilogy. The film starts in Philadelphia where a zombie pandemic is taking place and the situation is getting out of control. Francine and Stephen work in TV studios and are planning to steal a helicopter to escape from the zombies. In the meantime a SWAT team has laid siege to a building where the residents refuse to deliver the living dead – as their bodies belong to their loved ones. Roger and Peter are among the SWAT team members. They meet in the building and Roger tells Peter about the plan to escape in the helicopter together with Stephen and Francine.

The four end up going to one of the newly built indoor malls and are able to build a place to call home. Peter is from Trinidad and talks about a voodoo priest who mentioned a prophecy that when there's no more room in hell the dead would start to walk the world. While in the mall, they often have to do clean-up operations to kill zombies and prevent them from forcing their way in en masse. At first they enjoy their lifestyle but soon they start to feel imprisoned in the mall. In one operation, Roger is bitten and eventually turns into a zombie. Francine becomes pregnant, but Stephen tries to persuade her to have an abortion. At some point they talk about leaving but Stephen is opposed. Eventually a group of bikers enters the mall and a gun battle starts. Stephen is shot in the arm and bitten by multiple zombies in an elevator. Once reanimated as a zombie, he is able to remember how to lead the zombies to Francine and Peter. Both escape to the helicopter, Francine goes first and wants to escape but Peter contemplates suicide knowing that civilization has collapsed. In the end though he decides to escape with Francine in the helicopter. The world is collapsing and the future is uncertain.

Dawn of the Dead has an existentialist approach to life and civilization. Certainly, a collapse of civilization and extinction of the human race is possible. In fact, some people believe that extinction is our most likely fate. Knowing what has happened to civilization, Peter seriously considers suicide. Though great philosophers, such as Arthur Schopenhauer, state that suicide is a legitimate right, most humans tend to have an innate will to live no matter how bad the world or one's life has become. Following his survival instincts, Peter resists the urge to end his life with the goal of living as long as he can. The mall is the perfect setting for an existential reflection. Similarly to Sisyphus, the zombies live in a meaningless universe, wandering purposelessly from one side to the other of the mall, driven by mere instinct. A point can be made that in real life humans in malls are not much different from the zombies of *Dawn of the Dead*.

In *Day of the Dead* (1985), a zombie apocalypse has already taken place. Dr. Sarah Bowman, a small group of scientists and a crew of soldiers led by Captain Henry Rhodes hunt zombies for scientific research at the same time as they attempt to look for any other humans in a world invaded by zombies. Dr. Logan – portrayed as a mad scientist – nicknamed Dr. Frankenstein by Rhodes, believes zombies can be retrained. For him, zombies have a problem in their limbic system (an anatomical area of the brain that regulate emotion and behavior) and their behaviors are driven by the R-Complex, also known as the reptilian brain (mainly the basal ganglia: caudate nucleus, putamen, globus pallidus, amygdala, thalamus, etc.). For Dr. Logan, as a result of this problem with the limbic system zombies are unable to regulate their emotions, and function at a very instinctual level. Dr. Logan believes, however, that zombies can be the subject of cognitive rehabilitation. He has used behavioral therapy principles like reward, positive reinforcement and time out techniques and has been able to make significant progress with Bub, a zombie who has reacquired some of his lost cognitive skills. Bub has gradually relearned how to use some tools such as a pistol and a record player. In addition, Bub has begun to show more prosocial behaviors, and he is able to integrate information. For instance, after seeing Rhodes he salutes him like a soldier. Rhodes, however, has no patience and kills Logan after discovering he is using human flesh from his dead soldiers as a food reward as part of his

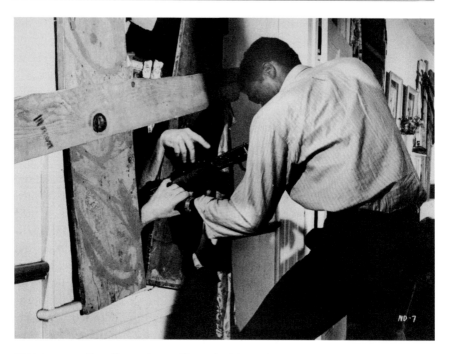

FIGURE 11.2 Ben Struggles to Keep the Living Dead out of the House (*Night of the Living Dead*)

therapy with Bub. The zombie becomes emotional and mourns the death of his master Dr. Logan once he finds his body.

The behavioral therapeutic skills portrayed in the film are accurate. Positive reinforcement of good behavior with the use of rewards is key in parental and behavioral skill training with children and adolescents who have emotional and behavioral disturbances. These techniques are also very useful in the coaching of humans and pets or other domestic animals. As depicted in *Day of the Dead*, cognitive rehabilitation often involves the use of the music they used to hear before losing their skills. This type of music therapy is used in people with cortical dementia such as Alzheimer's disease. The cognitive and behavior techniques shown in the film are also an essential in the treatment of autistic disorder with the goal of improving cognition and social behavior. Applied behavioral analysis (ABA) therapy, the latest treatment in autism, involves the use of reward and positive reinforcement to enhance cognition and social behavior. In *Day of the Dead*, Romero portrays a world in which humans can be more harmful than evil zombies.

Romero's latest film, *Land of the Dead* (2005), portrays a world in which humans and zombies have somehow learned to coexist. However, the humans live in a protected area of the city with clearly delimited social classes.

Humans seem to have momentarily taken control over the zombies and do as they wish. Some groups take expeditions to the zombie world in search of food, medicines and liquor. The crisis starts when an African American zombie known as Big Daddy begins to naturally recover cognitive and emotional skills. He gets frustrated by the dehumanizing way the living treat the dead and leads a group of zombies to the city to fight back. In the city, a few wealthy ambitious men are building an exclusive high-rise area called Fiddler's Green. However, Big Daddy leads his people across the river to maul all the wealthy people living there.

Land of the Dead reflects on the financial crisis and the disparities in this world. An African American zombie takes over and makes the changes needed. This has interesting parallels with the rise of Obama to power in the United States. Furthermore the film reflects on human nature, as the living have been able to control the zombie epidemics and now seem to be in control. Now instead humans are abusing the zombies. Zombies are killed for mere fun, and they are used for games and excitement in clubs. In *Land of the Dead*, the victims have already become the abusers. Zombies are now able to recuperate some of their lost cognitive skills spontaneously, something that brings hope for a zombie existence. In fact Cholo, one of the characters, decides not to kill himself once bitten by a zombie in order to explore living on the other side.

Romero's zombies greatly influenced the *Resident Evil* film franchise (2002–2012, with one due in 2017) by Paul Anderson. In this series, a corporation called Umbrella controls healthcare, research and insurances without the awareness of the population. A toxic substance that turns the employees into zombies is released. The system tries to control the plague but is unsuccessful.

Steven Schlozman, M.D. (a psychiatrist at Massachusetts General Hospital and friend of George Romero) wrote a book titled *The Zombie Autopsies*. The book's narrative will be the basis of George Romero's next zombie film. For Schlozman, zombies can be approached neuroscientifically. For instance, zombies lack ability for executive function (the ability to plan ahead), as they seem impulsive and driven by their most primary needs. This can be explained by abnormalities in the prefrontal cortex of the brain. At the same time, their uncoordinated gait, also known as ataxic gait, could be explained by abnormalities in their cerebellum, while their constant hunger might be due to a problem in their hypothalamus, the area in the brain that signals hunger and satiation.

After *Night of the Living Dead*, writer John Russo retained the rights to all of his *Living Dead* titles. He wrote the original script for the movie *The Return of the Living Dead* (1985). Director David O'Bannon agreed to direct the movie on the condition that he could modify the script towards a dark comedy with a punk atmosphere and aesthetic style, congruent with the trends of the time. In fact, The Cramps were commissioned to produce the soundtrack among other punk artists.

The film also starts from the position of post-atomic era paranoia as it concerns experiments done by the government that have resulted in a very hazardous substance. In the film, Frank introduces his new employee, Freddy, to the routine of his new job in a company that sells medical products. Frank shows him a container with the toxic substance and Freddy accidentally breaks it, making the two fall unconscious. The substance reanimates one of the dead bodies preserved for anatomy lectures. Frank and Freddy take the body to the mortuary to burn and destroy it but this causes the release of the toxic substance into the air and creates an acid rain that reanimates the dead. This scene has some parallels with the rain that came after the atomic bomb in Hiroshima. A different interpretation might be a potential parallel with lysergic acid (LSD), which was used by the government as well for secret experiments of mind control.

The film approaches interesting aspects in the study of consciousness. Frank and Freddy are dying due to the toxic effects of the substance but retain full consciousness. Some neurodegenerative conditions like amyotrophic lateral sclerosis can present similarly. Freddy resists accepting his fatal fate and shows ambivalence when the physician informs him that he already has rigor mortis, the muscle rigidity that characterizes the dead. In this film, the concept of zombies hungry for brains rather than flesh is introduced. In addition, zombies retain awareness of their status as dead, and eating brains from the living seems therapeutic. In one scene, a female zombie, who preserves only her body above the waist, is captured after eating the brain of one of the protagonists. The zombie tells the protagonists that she eats brains to relieve the pain of being dead.

In consciousness studies, a philosophical zombie or p-zombie is a hypothetical being indistinguishable from a human except by the fact that it lacks consciousness. Zombie arguments support the notion that p-zombies are possible in a mind–body dualistic approach to consciousness. According to a dualistic model, humans have both physical properties (body or weight) and mental properties (consciousness, intentionality, and a sense of self). By contrast, physicalism is the thesis that everything is physical, or that everything is consequent to the physical. In physicalism, the nature of the actual world conforms, to a certain point, the condition of being physical. While supporters of mind–body dualism argue that p-zombies are possible, physicalists insist that at some point the mind will have a physical matter. Therefore, physicalists believe that p-zombies are impossible. Over the last few decades, psychiatry has gradually switched from a dualistic to a physicalist approach. Many scholars now believe that all human behavior has at the end of the day some neurochemical or neurogenetic explanation. In that case, p-zombies would not be compatible with current psychiatric thinking and the only possibility of conceptualizing p-zombies would be by conceiving an entire zombie human existence.

While Romero's and Russo's zombies become reanimated as the result of radioactivity or toxic substances, over the last two decades most zombie films have established an infectious etiology for zombie transformation. For instance, author Max Brooks affirms in his *Zombie Survival Guide* that zombie states are caused by infection with a "solanum," a virus traveling through the bloodstream, from the initial point of entry – usually the bite site – to the brain, causing encephalitis. For Brooks, a solanum would in a mysterious way use frontal lobe neurons for replication, causing its destruction. This would explain how zombies have no ability for planning – the so-called executive function – which surrenders them to their most primitive instincts. Once infected with solanum the person experiences fever, sweats, pain, discoloration and gradual cessation of all bodily functions causing cardiac and respiratory failure and death but leaving the brain in a coma, while the virus mutates its cells into a completely new organ.

An example of this kind of brain zombie infection is portrayed in Danny Boyle's film *28 Days Later* (2002). Similarly to Romero's *Living Dead* series, the film is set in a post-apocalyptic world that is the result of a zombie pandemic. Here investigations with chimpanzees in Cambridge, UK result in a rage-inducing virus. A group of three animal rights activists release the chimpanzees, spreading the infection worldwide. Jim, the main character, wakes up in the hospital after a prolonged coma without knowing what has happened. Wandering around in the streets of London, he is attacked by a group of infected people but is rescued by Selena. Later they meet Frank and his daughter Hannah and travel in search of a military refuge. However, the army turns out to be even more dangerous than the infected.

The rage virus portrayed in *28 Days Later* seems inspired by the rabies infection. Rabies is a disease caused by a type of *Lyssavirus* with a reservoir in bats, dogs and monkeys – as in the film – and raccoons or coyotes. This virus causes inflammation in the brain and salivary glands, salivation, anxiety, and agitation, causing biting as well as refusal of water or liquids. As with how people are said to be turned into zombies, the virus can be transmitted through the saliva by biting and inoculation in the bloodstream.

The successful TV show *The Walking Dead* (2010–) and the film *28 Days Later* are both inspired by the same comic, also titled *The Walking Dead*. In the TV show Rick Grimes also wakes up in hospital after a coma without knowing about the pandemics. He walks alone in the streets of Atlanta until being attacked by a group of zombies. He is rescued by a group of survivors that takes him to a camp where he encounters his wife, son and old friend.

Boyle was the executive producer of the sequel *28 Weeks Later* (2007). For that he commissioned Spanish director Juan Carlos Fresnadillo. The sequel is also set in London. In the film, Don and his wife Alice hide in a country house with a group of people trying to escape the infection but they are attacked by a group of the infected. They are about to escape but army medical officer Scarlet returns to save one child who is hiding in the wardrobe when the infected arrive. Full of fear, Don leaves his wife and the child behind and manages to escape. Twenty-eight weeks later, the infected have died of hunger and the UK is officially free of disease.

Don's children, who were in the United States during the epidemic, return to their country, now controlled by the military. As they reunite with their father, they are curious about the circumstances in which their mother died. Don is still conflicted by guilt and shame about what he did and distorts the story. However, his wife is found alive and apparently asymptomatic in the house. She is found to be infected and a carrier but somehow immune to the infection. Don visits her to ask for forgiveness and when she tells him that she loves him, he kisses her, becoming infected with the rage virus. Under this rage syndrome, Don kills his wife and spreads the infection again. The situation gets out of control and the military begins to take radical measures. Don has an idea of how to reunite the family in a different way.

The most significant psychological moment in the film happens at the beginning when Don impulsively abandons his wife to save his life. Under acute stress when someone's life is threatened a fight, flight or freeze instinctual response has been key in the survival of our species for millennia. In this case, Don saves his life by fleeing without thinking. It is a survival instinct that operates without thinking or planning. However, once he gets time to reflect on what he did, an overwhelming feeling of guilt becomes prominent and he gradually develops a fantasy that he did everything he could, in order to cope with it. He shares this modified version of the story with his children and that the more he repeats it, the more real it becomes.

REC (2007) is a Spanish movie directed by Jaume Balagueró and Paco Plaza. It was shot as a found footage film and describes a first outbreak zombie infection in a residential building of Barcelona. In the first scene, reporter Angela is doing a program for a night show about the routine of firefighters. While filming the show, the firefighters get a call from a building where an older lady has been screaming insanely. Apparently a dog has transmitted a virus to a little girl and some of the neighbors. It turns out that the infection had originated years earlier when a little girl from Portugal known as *La Niña Medeiros* began to show signs of possession. The church had intervened but the infection was in fact the result of an enzyme that could mutate and so went out of control. Angela and the cameraman learn about this after finding a tape recorder in an abandoned apartment of the building where La Niña Medeiros has been living all these years.

Balagueró and Plaza combine demonic possession and zombie infection in this film. However, the film concludes that an enzyme, likely an infective protein, causes the disease. In microbiology, infective proteins that lack DNA or RNA to qualify as viruses are known as prions. The most well-known prion disease is spongiform encephalopathy (mad cow disease), which can be transmitted to humans through the ingestion of meat contaminated with the prion.

World War Z is an apocalyptic horror novel that narrates the accounts of a United Nations agent following a devastating zombie pandemic worldwide. The novel was adapted into a successful motion film (2013) directed by Marc Foster and produced by and starring Brad Pitt. In the film, the key to survival is to be sick. The infected look for healthy prey and instinctively skip sick people; this leads to research focused on the development of a vaccine that does not affect humans and keeps the infected uninterested.

The success of zombie culture can be approached sociologically. A zombie epidemic results in chaos, anarchy and the abolition of the current system. Society may regress to its most primitive form, in which survival is the major goal. Nevertheless the modern zombie is not the result of Haitian folklore, slavery and colonialism. Romero was not inspired by the first Hollywood voodoo zombies. The modern zombie inherits the collective anxiety about the plagues and other calamities that have affected Western history such as the collective unconscious fear of rabies as the disease is transmitted in the saliva through bites, the fear of leprosy since zombies are walking bodies with parts that fall off in different states of decomposition, and the fear of devastating plagues. Throughout the centuries, human beings have suffered severe pandemics that threatened extinction, the most prominent example being that of the Black Death, which took place between 1346 and 1353 in Europe, taking the lives of nearly two-thirds of the European population. Romero's zombie collects all these Western fears of the Apocalypse, a central theme in European history, with the artistic images of *memento mori* (reflection on mortality) and the Danse Macabre (or Dance of Death, an allegory of the universality of death). The modern zombie is also related to the vampiric legends about the undead. Historically, multiple threats have put our species in danger of extinction. Perhaps the most recent example is World War II and the discovery of nuclear energy. Nowadays, a severe financial crisis in our capitalistic society has tested the entire system, causing ruin and devastation and a good deal of uncertainty. In times of societal crisis, apocalyptic horror cinema provides cathartic relief to audiences.

CHAPTER 12

Body Horror

BODY HORROR IS A specific subgenre of horror film in which the body becomes the subject of terror. Mutilation, disintegration, transformation and parasitism are common themes in body horror. Body art departed from Jackson Pollock's action painting and used the artist's own body for artistic expression. Often these expressions were performances and video recordings that involved self-harm, mutilation, masochism and intoxication. One of the first artists in this movement was Frenchman Yves Klein who, contrary to American Expressionist artists who were interested in expressing their personalities on the canvas, purported to express spirituality through the monochrome of the color blue. In one of his performances called *Living Brush* (1960), he asked a group of women to paint their torsos in blue before falling on a canvas and leaving their body print. The same year, he became interested in the subjects of telepathy and levitation. He had a picture taken of himself jumping from a two-story building published in his one-day journal that was distributed through all newsstands in Paris.

Viennese Actionism in Europe and several artists in the United States took body art to its fullest expression. Vito Acconci in *Seedbed* (1971) lay underneath a gallery masturbating and sharing his sexual fantasies with the visitors. Marina Abramović in *Rhythm 0* (1974) allowed visitors to touch her, mutilate her, and paint on her for six hours during a performance. The same year, Chris Burden had himself crucified on a Volkswagen Beetle. Bob Flanagan, an artist who suffered from cystic fibrosis, expressed his art through acts of masochism. In his performance *Auto-erotic SM* (1989) he carried out a number of masochistic acts with his partner. The act concluded with Flanagan nailing his penis onto a wooden board.

In 1977 David Lynch directed his debut film *Eraserhead* supported by the American Film Institute. Its main protagonist is Henry, a middle-aged man with a Frankenstein's bride-like hairdo. As he is about to enter his apartment with the groceries, his neighbor tells him that he has been invited by his girlfriend Mary and his parents for dinner. Once at the dinner, Mary's talkative father asks him to cut the chicken. However, the chicken seems to be moving and releases some gross substance. Mary leaves the room nauseated and her mother follows her. When they return to the living room, Mary's mother confronts Henry and, while trying to kiss him, asks Henry if he has had intercourse with her daughter. Henry doesn't answer but Mary is pregnant and his paternity is presumed. After the child is born Mary and Henry begin taking care of their reptilian-like baby in his apartment. However, frustrated with her inability to take care of him, Mary leaves Henry with the baby. Alone with the baby, Henry starts to have some visions and dreams of a childish lady in the radiator who dances and steps on big spermatozoids which are also ejected from his girlfriend's vagina. In one scene his baby grows inside from the neck ejecting his head into a pool and subsequently into the sky and the street. As it crashes, the cranium opens leaving the brain exposed. Next a boy in the street finds the head and takes it to a pencil factory to be turned into erasers. In a subsequent scene, Henry opens the bandages of his crying baby, which results in his organs spreading on the table. He decides to cut the baby's heart with scissors to alleviate his suffering. In the final scene the lady in the radiator embraces Henry as silence follows.

For Lynch, the film is about the darkness and confusion that there is in all of us. The film's surrealistic scenes are reminiscent of Luis Buñuel's *Un Chien Andalou* (1929). The cinematography has influenced other films such as Darren Aronofsky's *Pi* (1998). Psychiatrically, Henry's hallucinations happen in times between falling asleep and waking up, something known as hypnagogic and hypnopompic hallucinations. These types of hallucinations happen in all of us and are not considered pathological. However, in Henry's case, the confusion progresses to a more permanent level.

Henry seems to have poor support and poor social skills, and when left alone with the baby his anxiety rises to an almost psychotic level. His visual hallucinations could also be a symptom of conversion disorder, a syndrome characterized by neurological symptoms without organic explanation and generally thought to be related to anxiety. However, in the director's words, *Eraserhead* is a film about confusion and darkness. Henry is left alone in his small apartment with a deformed baby who gets sick with some kind of virus and cries all day. Due to this he barely sleeps and does not drink or eat properly. Henry begins to have difficulties differentiating what is real and what's not. In this context, the picture may well depict a case of delirium, an acute confusional state that results from disease; prolonged isolation; lack of stimulation; and inappropriate sleep, hydration or nutrition. Henry's confusion presents acutely in an already middle-aged man and progresses with his inability to handle the situation. Visual rather than auditory hallucinations, together with an inability to integrate information, fluctuating consciousness, purposeless behavior and disorganized thinking as depicted here would be suggestive of a delirium diagnosis.

Eraserhead was released to small audiences but soon gained a cult status. Two years after, Ridley Scott directed *Alien* (1979) based on a story by Dan O'Bannon about a group of astronauts in stasis that is unexpectedly awakened by the system of their craft after receiving a signal from a planetoid. As they arrive there, they find a spacecraft with the remains of a large alien that seems to have exploded. Executive Officer Kane finds a room full of eggs. As he inspects one of the eggs, a creature pops up from inside, attaches strongly to his face and leaves him in a coma. They plan to carry Kane back to re-enter their spacecraft but this violates quarantine rules. Warrant Officer Ripley tries to stop them but her efforts are thwarted by Ash, one of the scientists. In an attempt to detach the parasite from Kane's face, the crew finds that its blood is so corrosive that the craft would be in danger if they cut it. Eventually the parasite leaves the face and dies, but later, a small alien bursts from Kane's chest and escapes. The crew finds out that Ash was an android and was following instructions to bring the creature alive to Earth. The alien starts kidnapping the members of the crew one by one to use them as hosts for future reproduction but Ripley manages to thwart the creature's plans and throw it away from the craft, possibly saving humanity.

Alien is highly influenced by the Cold War films of the 1950s, in particular by *The Thing from Another World* (1951), *Invasion of the Body Snatchers* and *Forbidden Planet*. The film, however, was released in the context of the end of the Cold War and the oil crisis of 1979. Still, a fear of invasion remained in society. *Alien*'s major contribution to body horror is the fear of mutilation, and disintegration of one's body as a result of an infective parasite. The creature attaches to Kane's body, and uses his body for reproduction.

In real life, humans have dealt with parasites that threatened our lives. For instance, taenias are parasitic tapeworms that infect human intestines after consumption of its eggs in the intermediate host – usually pigs and cattle. Though the prevalence of taeniasis is low in developed countries, a collective fear of this kind of parasitism still remains. Furthermore the film raises important questions about human evolution and survival. The alien is portrayed as an evil creature but in fact it is just attempting to survive and possibly spread its species. In that sense, this alien species is not different from us. In this case, the film portrays a failed attempt to conquer our planet but lights the way to what most scientists propose as our best survival chance: to expand and conquer other planets and use their resources.

The film also comments on the fear of technology through the character of Ash, an android that is indistinguishable from the other humans and almost causes the destruction of humanity. Nevertheless Ash just follows commands from other humans. The question of whether Ash has consciousness or not remains open. Following his decapitation and right before his incineration, Ash makes a cynical comment about the crew's survival chances, something unlikely to have been programmed and more supportive of the theory of an android with consciousness. This aspect is a core theme of Scott's later film *Blade Runner* (1982).

Ridley Scott's prequel *Prometheus* (2012) came more than thirty years after a few sequels. According to Greek mythology, Prometheus was a Greek Titan who was punished by the gods after giving man the gift of fire without their approval. In Scott's film, a crew takes an expedition to a planet in the search of the Creator with the hope of getting a response to the eternal questions of our existence. As in real life, the questions in the film go for the most part unanswered, congruent with the more modern existential philosophical approaches of Western culture.

The peak period for body horror came during the 1980s. In 1980, Ken Russell directed *Altered States*. In the film Edward Jessup is a Harvard scientist of abnormal psychology who studies schizophrenia. Using an isolation tank, he explores other states of consciousness with the use of psychedelic substances. His experiments result in a gradual devolution of his humanity into a more primitive man. *Altered States* combines elements of psychedelia with body art and horror. The film was directed by Ken Russell based on the novel (1978) of the same name by Paddy Chayefsky who also wrote the screenplay for the film. The story is inspired by the research experiments of John Lilly who devised the first isolation tank in 1954 at the National Institute of Mental Health. Lilly was a physician and a psychoanalyst who graduated from and trained at the University of Pennsylvania. Lilly made major contributions to neuroscience. A major area of his research focused on exploring if communication between humans and dolphins was possible. In the 60s, he experimented with LSD and other psychedelic drugs in isolation tanks. In his book *The Center of the Cyclone*, he narrated his experiences transcending the limits of the mind by taking psychedelics in isolation tanks.

In *Altered States*, Dr. Edward Jessup is a researcher at Weill Cornell Medical College. He has done several experiments with his students in isolation tanks. Dr. Jessup has found that most of them find the experience pleasant and exhilarating, and some of them hallucinate. Dr. Jessup decides to try the isolation tank himself and discovers that he has multiple religious hallucinations, most of them about the Book of Revelation. Jessup is interested in researching intrinsic religious experiences. After meeting Emily, a Ph.D. student from Columbia, he explains that religion seems very important in people with schizophrenia and that is the reason he works with this population. With the isolation tank he believes he can reproduce the schizophrenic experience. While making love with Emily for first time, he has a mystical experience and starts thinking of Jesus and the Crucifixion. In that moment he tells Emily that he lost his faith when he was sixteen years old. At that time his father, whom he admired very much, contracted cancer. He used to take care of him daily and his father spent his last week of life in a coma. His last words were "terrible, terrible." After that experience, Jessup came to the realization that even for good humans like his father, the purpose of all suffering is just more suffering.

Jessup and Emily eventually marry and have children, both of them move to Boston to work at Harvard but Jessup does not feel fulfilled with that kind of conventional life and they eventually split. Jessup believes that the Self, the individual mind, and not God, contains immortality and the ultimate Truth. For him the atoms from which we are formed are six billion years old and contain the energy of the mind. Jessup is committed to finding the path to an earlier state of consciousness that can explain the meaningless horror in our lives. Jessup goes with his friend Eduardo Echeverría to Mexico to assist in a ceremony of indigenous people involving a shared hallucinatory experience. Apparently the drug used in the ceremony can be helpful in evoking ancient memories. The shaman advises Jessup that there will be a break and out of that break, his unborn soul will come out of the nothingness. During the ceremony, Jessup is asked to drink his blood mixed with natural psychedelics and in an altered consciousness state he kills a lizard. Jessup takes some of these powerful psychedelics with him to Boston and continues his experiments in the isolation tank at Harvard. Eventually he begins to experience biological devolution to more primitive human forms and in subsequent experiments he regresses to conscious primordial matter. Only the love of his wife can save him. Jessup discovers that the final Truth is that there is no final Truth.

Dr. Jessup's initial research focuses on the relationship between religiosity and schizophrenia. In an article written for the journal *Transcultural Psychiatry* in 2011, Simon Dein and Roland Littlewood argue that religion and psychosis have had a related evolutionary trajectory. Iconographically, many of Jessup's hallucinations are related to the Book of Revelation, the last book of the Bible written by a certain John on the island of Patmos, in the Aegean Sea. Though tradition has credited the writer of the Apocalypse, the writer of The Gospel and Jesus's disciple as being one and the same John, now it is accepted that these were three different persons. The name "Apocalypse" comes from the Greek *apocalypsis*, which means unveiling or revelation, hence the English name "Book of Revelation." Some of the most popular images of medieval art are based on the Book of Revelation such as the Last Judgment. In addition, it contains a series of phantasmagorical events that hypothetically will take place at the end of times. For example, the book states that after the Lamb with seven eyes and seven horns opens the book with the seven seals, the four horsemen will start their battle; one of them is Death who will kill everyone on Earth with the sword, hunger and disease. This scene is depicted in one of Dr. Jessup's hallucinatory experiences.

Psychedelic drugs, whether natural such as psilocybin, peyote, belladonna or synthetic like LSD, are thought to cause their effect through serotonin agonism at the 5-HT2A receptor. However, the drug that Jessup takes in Mexico seems to be ayahuasca, which is the result of a brew of a plant named

Banisteriopsis caapi. Though not fully understood, in contrast to other psychedelics, ayahuasca's hallucinogenic mechanism is explained by inhibition of monoamine oxidase, an enzyme that metabolizes the neurotransmitter norepinephrine. Ayahuasca can increase the heart rate and pressure and cause vomiting and diarrhea, something that has been thought helpful by South American natives in the elimination of parasites. Ayahuasca was already being used by indigenous people in Peru at the time the first Spaniards arrived. However, as compared to other psychedelics, ayahuasca has gone through a recent revival in popularity in Western countries. This might be partially related to its short-acting strong psychedelic effects and the relatively "trendy" shamanistic ritual around its use.

In *Altered States*, Jessup goes to Mexico to find more powerful drugs with the hope of making some progress with his research about different states of human consciousness since his experiments in the isolation tank are not fruitful. Mathematician and philosopher David Chalmers notes that today, despite an explosion in the numbers of consciousness studies, we still cannot connect structure to function. In trying to unveil "radically" a theory of consciousness Chambers suggests making consciousness a fundamental building block of the universe (like gravity, space, time, mass, and charge). Moreover, he proposes that consciousness is pan-psychic; that's to say consciousness is universal and made of elementary particles which are primitive precursors of consciousness. Thus consciousness becomes a continuum between mind and nature. Jessup also explains a similar thesis in *Altered States*, as for him the atoms that form our body are at least six billion years old. He believes his experiments will take him to the original moment of the Self.

After experimenting with the new drug, Jessup devolves towards an ancient human, supposedly an earlier state of consciousness. Psychologist Julian Jaynes explains that 1,000 years BCE, humans likely did not have a conscious awareness of the self in the way we have today. For him this would be explained by the evolution from a bicameral (the two sides of the brain working independently) to a unicameral brain (the two sides working conjointly). For Jaynes, ancient humans functioned by means of automatic, non-conscious habits like other animals. Jaynes explains that the hallucinations in schizophrenia could also be the result of a brain functioning in a bicameral way. While it is possible that the origins of human consciousness are explained by Jaynes's theory, it is unlikely that self-awareness arose only 3,000 years ago as the earliest cave paintings have been dated from 41,000 years ago. These paintings consist of hand stencils, and the level of cognitive sophistication needed to leave a hand stencil would imply a high likelihood of self-awareness. It is likely that already by that time humans had developed a theory of mind; that is to say the ability to attribute mental states to oneself and others. Nonetheless, animal consciousness might be better explained in a spectrum rather than a dichotomic human versus non-human animal model.

Though a good explanatory model of consciousness is still lacking, the spectrum model proposes that most animals have some form of consciousness. A number of scientists argue that monkeys, dolphins and parrots have consciousness in similar way as humans. At the other end of the spectrum would be less sophisticated animal structures such as jellyfish or worms. Today, even some neurobiologists argue that though not self-conscious, plants also have intelligence and consciousness.

Altered States explores the subject of biological devolution to a more basic and primitive state of human consciousness. Jessup plays God in the search for the absolute Truth to discover that there is no absolute Truth or, at least, that we do not have the tools to determine it.

John Carpenter's remake of *The Thing* and Wes Craven's *A Nightmare on Elm Street* are also good examples of body horror masterpieces. In 1985 Stuart Gordon directed *Re-animator* based on a novella by H.P. Lovecraft. It tells the story of Herbert West, a medical student at the University of Zurich who has created a substance that allows dead people to come back to life. In the first scene West has given life to one of his respected professors Dr. Gruber, but the results aren't as expected. After this, West travels to the United States to study at Miskatonic University in New England. There he meets Dr. Hill, a brain researcher and neurosurgeon interested in the discovery of the brain's anatomical region responsible for human will. West accuses him of copying Gruber's ideas.

West moves in with Dan, a medical student who is dating his classmate Megan, the daughter of Dr. Halsey, the dean of the medical school. While in Dan's apartment, he starts his own lab in his room in the basement. When Dan's cat Rufus is killed on the road West reanimates him with the reagent. Despite Rufus coming back an aggressive cat, Dan believes in the therapeutic possibilities of this substance. Dan tries to explain the potential of the reagent to Dr. Halsey but he believes West and Dan have gone mad and bars them both from the medical school. Later Dan and West go to the morgue to resuscitate a dead body and prove their thesis but after reanimating the body, Dr. Halsey arrives on the scene and gets killed by an animated corpse. Then, West and Dan inject the reagent into Halsey who comes back to life as a zombie. Thinking that Halsey has suffered a mental breakdown, Dr. Hill takes care of him and treats him with a lobotomy. However, he soon discovers Halsey is a reanimated corpse and starts blackmailing West so that he discloses the secret formula of the reagent. Feeling that Hill is trying to take ownership of his discovery, West decapitates him and reanimates him afterwards. A decapitated Hill knocks West out, steals his reagent with the notes and kidnaps Megan for his experiments. West and Dan rescue Megan but Hill is now able to control other reanimated corpses with his mind. West injects Hill with a lethal dose of reagent but instead he mutates and becomes more dangerous. During the altercation between West and Hill, Dan and Megan try to escape but she is lethally attacked by a corpse. The film ends with a scream after Dan reanimates Megan.

Through the centuries, humans have attempted to beat mortality with the use of alchemy and a number of magical remedies. West here embodies the mad scientist archetype. However, he is good-hearted and motivated by the cause of advancing science. The film concludes that if we challenge the rules of nature, the consequences can be devastating. In many ways, the films reminds us of *Frankenstein*, in which a scientist is motivated to decipher the secret of mortality and the discovery of a mechanism to bring the dead back to life. Dr. Hill reminds us of Dr. Mabuse; he also has an ability to control others' minds telepathically. Moreover he is obsessed with the discovery of the anatomy of the will. However, Hill's experiments don't lead to the expected results and instead he borrows ideas from others, Gruber's initially and West's later. The anatomy of the will is still in debate in the domains of neuroscience. While consciousness has long been attributed to the cerebral cortex, the ability to plan in life and make decisions has been especially related to the prefrontal cortex – the so-called executive function capacity. A recent publication by Sam Harris called *Free Will* (2012) proposes that electroencephalogram studies probe the existence of subcortical electrical activity before any sign in the cortex; in other words our intention is unconscious prior to becoming a conscious thought. Harris explains that if human behavior is anticipated by subcortical structures, free will would not therefore be possible. That is to say there would be no freedom, or at least, not in the way we have traditionally understood it. However, even today it is difficult to establish such a binary model of cortical conscious will versus subcortical unconscious behavior. In psychiatry, especially in the realms of psychotherapy, space for an at least partial will – the so-called compatibilist model – is needed. In psychoanalytic therapy, one can through free association of random thoughts and dreams become aware of the unconscious drives and memories that play a role in our actions that could therefore become the subject of conscious manipulation. In cognitive psychotherapy patients become aware of cognitive distortions and negative thoughts that result in bad emotions and reactions. For example, through cognitive exercises and homework assignments a patient will practice alternative behaviors that will shape their emotions and behaviors. Although it's an abstract concept, in the lack of a better construct, free will serves society. Perhaps a pragmatic approach to free will is the most reasonable in the present time.

The year after the release and success of *Re-animator* Stuart Gordon directed *From Beyond* (1986) which was also loosely based on a short story by H.P. Lovecraft of the same name. In the film, Dr. Edward Pretorius and his assistant Crawford have created a machine called the resonator that stimulates the pineal gland with the goal of helping to reach a new dimension. When activated a creature appears and subsequently decapitates Pretorius.

The authorities find Crawford is presumably guilty and insane and he is confined to a psychiatric hospital. There he is seen by Dr. Katherine McMichaels, a young psychiatrist with a more modern approach. Crawford explains the circumstances of Pretorius's death and their experiments with the resonator and the pineal gland. Katherine is left with a gut feeling that there could be some truth in Crawford's claims and orders a CT scan of the head, which shows an enlargement of the pineal gland. Consequently she convinces the team to go with Crawford and Detective Bubba Brownlee back to the house and activate the resonator. There they learn about Pretorius's sadomasochistic fantasies. After activating the resonator new creatures come out and a grossly deformed evil Pretorius with special powers appears from the new dimension. Katherine, however, continues to be interested in the resonator despite Crawford's warning as she believes this machine can lead to the discovery of a treatment for schizophrenia. She reactivates the resonator, which makes her hypersexual and releases new creatures. Bubba shuts off the power and when they are about to leave, Pretorius activates the resonator again. At that moment little bee-like creatures appear, which kill Bubba. Katherine manages to short-circuit the machine with an extinguisher and takes a sick Crawford back to the hospital. Now both are thought to be insane. Katherine is about to receive electroconvulsive therapy but the team stops as they learn that Crawford has escaped. Crawford's hypertrophic pineal gland makes him eat fresh brains from people and when he is about to try to do the same with Katherine she bites off his pineal gland, something that restores his sanity. Together they go back to the house to destroy the resonator with a bomb but Pretorius eats Crawford. Katherine, however, escapes as the bomb explodes.

Unlike *Re-animator's* West, Edward Pretorius portrays here an evil mad scientist. In Machiavellian fashion he will do whatever is needed to carry out his plan to reach a new dimension. He has fantasies of power and control. With this machine he pretends to become a new type of super human and gain the ability to control others. Pretorius has narcissistic and antisocial traits of personality disorder and has no empathy for others' fate. This is often referred as malignant narcissism. He is focused on his own goals and furthermore has sadistic fantasies (as evident in the number of sadomasochistic videos and toys found in his room). Sadism is usually considered a deviant sexual behavior driven by an internal need for control and oppression of the other, something that would corroborate the malignant narcissistic theory. Pretorius manipulates Crawford and makes him believe he is super intelligent.

In contrast, Katherine has altruistic motivations. Her brother had schizophrenia. Frustrated with her inability to save him she later became a psychiatrist. Psychologically, helplessness when a loved one becomes sick is a major reason for people to become health care professionals. Katherine likely felt that her brother received poor treatment. She is judgmental when talking about current psychiatric therapies and attempts to approach patients in what she thinks is a more humane and compassionate way. She is caring, compassionate and listens to them. Her thoughts are influenced by the ideas about psychiatry resulting from 1960s counterculture.

Pretorius and Crawford's experiments are centered on the pineal gland, a small endocrine gland in the brain located above the thalamus responsible for the production of melatonin, a hormone that regulates the sleep–wake cycle. As the film points out when Katherine and Crawford first meet, seventeenth-century philosopher René Descartes referred to the pineal gland as the third eye and the seat of the soul. Coincidentally or not, more recent research signals the pineal gland as the key organ in the production of endogenous psychedelics and a possible target of psychedelic drugs such as marijuana and N,N-Dimethyltryptamine (DMT). Psychedelics are thought to act as catalysts towards the exploration of different dimensions and transcendence.

The film explores the possibility of a new dimension that could take a person to live eternally. In philosophy, the four-dimension theory, eternalism or perdurantism, explores the idea that a subject exists independently of time and space. This theory contrasts with presentism, which gives existential credit to the present tense only. Congruent with an eternalist approach to existence, Pretorius is able to continue existing in a fourth dimension. With the help of the resonator he will be able to return to the three-dimensional world and carry out his malevolent plans.

Another film based on the existence of a new dimension of existence is *Hellraiser* (1987), a film written and directed by acclaimed horror director Clive Barker based on his own novella. The story starts somewhere in North Africa where Frank Cotton buys a puzzle box from a dealer. After solving the puzzle he is torn apart by swinging hooked chains which appear. In a different scene, Frank's brother Larry moves to his childhood house with his second wife Julia, who apparently had had an affair with Frank in the past. Larry cuts his hand with a nail while moving a couch and drips blood in the attic. The blood awakens Frank's body and he contacts Julia to convince her to bring him more people in order to drink their blood. Julia picks up men in bars for him and he drinks the blood of these men to regenerate his body. Frank then kills his own brother Larry to use his skin and escape with Julia. However, Frank is now more interested in his niece Kirsty who is younger and better looking. Kirsty escapes and finds the puzzle box, and after solving it she awakens the Cenobites who define themselves as explorers of the carnal experience that can no longer differentiate between pain and pleasure. They attempt to take Kirsty with them but she offers her uncle in exchange for her freedom.

The film depicts a typical case of a person with antisocial personality disorder, Frank Cotton. From the film we can infer that he has a history of failure to conform to social norms, and problems with authority. Due to the lack of excitement experienced in an antisocial personality, he will use harm, pain and violence to extremes in the search for pleasure. This involves stealing, an affair with his own brother's wife, and sadomasochism. He travels to Africa to get the puzzle box that will open the gate to a new dimension of pain and pleasure. Similarly to artist Bob Flanagan's masochistic performance, Frank ends up fatally mutilated by hooked chains.

One of the originators and most acclaimed directors of body horror is David Cronenberg. In his films he goes beyond the clear distinction of good and evil to deeper psychological and philosophical themes that involve the mutation and disintegration of one's body and mind. Two of his first films deal with the experiments of mad scientists; they create new toxic epidemics that threaten the populations – a repeated theme in later zombie films. In *Shivers* (1975) Dr. Emil Hobbes experiments with parasites to create substitutes for diseased body organs. However, these parasites turn people into maniacs. In *Rabid* (1977) surgeon Dan Keloid turns his patient into a vampire.

Cronenberg explored themes of telepathy, mind reading and telekinesis in *Scanners* (1981). In the film, a security company, for its own profitable purposes, attempts to use people referred to as "scanners," who have a type of supernatural gift. At the beginning of the film, the company shows a mind control experiment in which a scanner attempts to "read" a volunteer. The experiment goes wrong and the head of the volunteer explodes. This does not discourage the company from continuing to pursue their interest until a renegade scanner rebels against the company. *The Fly* (1986) was a remake of Kurt Neumann's classic with the same name (1958). Cronenberg's remake, however, focuses on the theme of witnessing the mutation of one's body and its psychological impact at a time in which science was making significant progress in the sequencing of DNA. *The Fly* narrates the story of Seth Brundle, a famous scientist who has designed a revolutionary teletransportation technique with the use of telepods. Veronica is a journalist for *Particle* magazine the editor of which is Veronica's former lover Stathis Borans. Veronica is assigned to write an article about Seth's scientific discoveries for the magazine. Seth shows her his new experiment. So far he has been successful in teletransporting inanimate objects but an earlier trial with a living being (a monkey) was catastrophic. Soon, Seth and Veronica begin a romantic relationship, which infuriates Borans who, driven by jealousy, decides to publish some of the secret information Seth had shared with Veronica. In the meantime, Seth manages to teletransport a baboon and later successfully tries the telepod on himself. After this, Seth realizes he is changing. He notices an unusual strength and other physical skills. Seth believes that these changes are related to purifying properties of the telepod but he starts to develop personality changes too. He becomes more arrogant and egocentric and accuses Veronica of being jealous of him. After his nails fall out, he understands there might be something wrong with him. Doing some research within his operating system, he discovers that a fly was in the telepod during his transportation and the system fused both Seth's and the fly's DNA.

Seth begins to metamorphose into something not human, a being that he calls Brundlefly. At that same time, Veronica realizes that she is pregnant and not knowing if she got pregnant before or after Seth's fusion with the fly, she asks Borans to help her arrange an abortion in the middle of the night. However, Brundlefly overheard the conversation during Veronica's last visit and abducts her before the abortion takes place. Borans follows them into the apartment and once he gets in, Brundlefly corrodes his hand and foot with his corrosive saliva. In that moment, Brundlefly reveals his plan to fuse Veronica, the baby and himself into a new being. However, right before his plan is about to be carried out, Borans is able to shoot at the cable leading to the telepod containing Veronica. Brundlefly then tries to escape his telepod but does not have enough time and the system fuses Brundlefly with parts of the telepod. Then, a new creature resulting from the fusion of Brundlefly, cables and metallic elements leaves the third telepod. At this moment, Brundlefly understands that he cannot live like this anymore and in a lucid moment of humanity gestures to Veronica to shoot him in the head. Veronica is initially hesitant but agrees to do it to alleviate her lover's suffering. She then crashes on the floor crying and grieving the death of her partner.

The tragic ending of *The Fly* is one of the most moving moments in the history of American cinema. The stories of Cronenberg's *The Fly* and Kafka's *The Metamorphosis* have interesting parallels. Similarly to Seth Brundle's story, in Kafka's novel, Gregor Samsa turns into a giant insect and has to learn how to live with his new nature to the consequent embarrassment of his family members. After he dies, his loved ones experience similar mixed feelings of grief and relief.

In the last few years Cronenberg has gradually shifted away from body horror to stories of overcoming difficulties in a hostile environment. *A History of Violence* (2005) and *Eastern Promises* (2007) are examples of this. In *A Dangerous Method* (2011), Cronenberg focuses on the history of psychoanalysis and the relationship between Eugen Bleuler and Sigmund Freud's pupil Carl Jung and Jung's patient and future analyst Sabina Spielrein.

Recently, Dutch director Tom Six has revived the interest in body horror with *The Human Centipede* (2009). In the film, Dr. Heiter, a mad German surgeon, kidnaps people to sew each to the next, anus to mouth, to create a human centipede. In the film's sequel (2011), Martin is the guard of a multistory car park and has an obsession with *The Human Centipede*. He watches the film constantly in his tollbooth at work and also has a pet centipede at home. His mother blames him for putting his father in prison after he sexually and physically abused Martin. His psychiatrist prescribes him medication and also touches him inappropriately. In this Dantesque environment, inspired by

Dr. Heiter, Martin's major goal in life becomes to make a much larger human centipede by kidnapping people in the parking lot. However, his surgical knowledge is non-existent and the results are disastrous.

CHAPTER 13

The Horror in the Asylum

PHILIPPE PINEL (1745–1826) WAS a French physician known for his advocacy and proposal of a more humane treatment of the mentally ill. Often credited as the man who freed the insane from their chains, he proposed a medical approach to mental illness. While working at La Salpêtrière in Paris, in 1798 he wrote *Nosographie philosophique ou La méthode de l'analyse appliquée à la médecine*, a manual that established the first classification of mental disorders. For Pinel mental diseases were classified in four different forms: melancholia, mania, dementia and idiocy. Furthermore, Pinel proposed a new therapy based on the creation of an asylum in which mentally ill patients could live in a community. This, according to Pinel, would gradually replace the prior treatments such as bloodletting, purging and physical restraints. Pinel's idea of an asylum included the same elements of any community in the outside world. Patients could work and participate in activities that form the principles of today's occupational therapy, and they could go to church. The hospital embraced the value of physical activity and socialization between patients to prepare them for reintroduction into society. The principles of moral treatment inspired William Tuke, in the York Retreat in England, and they subsequently spread to the United States. For instance, Rufus Wyman, the first superintendent of the Massachusetts Asylum for the Insane (renamed as McLean Hospital in 1823 after donations by John McLean) was a strong believer in moral treatment.

Moral treatment became the standard approach to mental illness throughout the nineteenth and first half of the twentieth century, a time in which new treatments were being developed. One of them was convulsive therapy. In 1927, Austrian psychiatrist Manfred Sakel used insulin to induce coma in patients as a result of hypoglycemia (low blood sugar) in their brains. This treatment showed a good short-term effect in patients with severe mental illness, once patients had recovered from the hypoglycemia. This treatment, however, carried significant risk and was gradually replaced by electroconvulsive therapy. Before the development of electroconvulsive therapy, in 1934,

Hungarian psychiatrist Ladislas Meduna proposed the use of a chemical called cardiazol to induce seizures in patients with severe mental conditions. Inspired by insulin shock therapy and cardiazol shock therapy, Italian neurologist Ugo Cerletti proposed instead the use of short-term electric current to induce convulsions after seeing significant improvement in a patient with delusions and hallucinations who returned to a normal state of mind in 1938. This new electroshock or electroconvulsive therapy was more practical and easy to apply and replaced chemical shock therapies.

In the first half of the twentieth century other physicians investigated the possibilities of surgical methods to treat mental illness. Portuguese neurosurgeon Egas Moniz believed that mental illness could be related to wrongful associations of neurons in the frontal lobes. He thought that a number of incisions in the white matter would allow the brain to heal and restore these "bad connections." With the help of neurosurgeon Pedro Lima he was able to inject ethanol into the subcortical white matter that connected the frontal lobe with other structures in a patient with melancholia (depression) in 1935. The operation was thought successful and they treated up to forty more patients who had melancholia, bipolar disorder, schizophrenia and obsessive-compulsive disorder. While these surgeries were restricted to a small number of patients, Walter Freeman in the United States conceived a method called transorbital lobotomy that consisted of accessing the frontal lobe through the orbit with the use of an icepick and a little hammer. Freeman proposed that his method was much simpler and lasted only a few minutes, thus it could be used after the short interval of anesthesia induced by electroshock therapy.

The popularity of electroconvulsive therapy and psychosurgical therapies declined with the discovery of neuroleptics (antipsychotics) and lithium as alternative chemical therapies for severe mental disorders. Moreover, in the 1960s, the so-called antipsychiatry movement challenged all the therapies at the time including asylum treatment, electroconvulsive therapy and psychosurgery. Several psychiatrists such as Franco Basaglia, Thomas Szasz, and David Cooper and sociologists like Michel Foucault among others challenged the conception of mental illness and argued that psychiatry served the government as an instrument for behavioral control. As a result, society disapproved of treatment in asylums and proposed the return of mentally ill patients to the community. This was also possible with the popularity of chlorpromazine and other psychopharmacological treatments that made outpatient treatment more feasible. This dramatic change in ideas about psychiatric treatment in a relatively short period of time was reflected in Ken Kesey's novel *One Flew over the Cuckoo's Nest*, which was adapted by Milos Forman to a motion picture in 1975. Though a great film, it unfairly depicts the use of electroconvulsive therapy and lobotomy as common methods used by psychiatrists – as suggested by an evil nurse – for punishment and behavior control.

Today, a number of psychiatrists and advocates of the mentally ill claim that the lack of support for inpatient or residential treatment has resulted in a significant increase of patients with mental illness ending up homeless or incarcerated in prisons. Electroconvulsive therapy is still a common treatment successful in patients with severe depression at risk for suicide who don't improve with standard psychopharmacological treatments. A therapy called transcranial magnetic stimulation, which also uses current on specific anatomical areas, is more practical and has little to no side effects, but it has not been proven to be as helpful as electroconvulsive therapy. While traditional psychosurgical treatments were abandoned due to their side effects (dysexecutive function syndrome, negative symptoms, emotional blunting, seizures and so on), studies using less invasive psychosurgical laser methods targeting specific structures (corpus callosum, amygdala, caudate or hippocampus) have been shown helpful in the treatment of severe obsessive-compulsive disorder and other severe conditions. Deep brain stimulation, a neurosurgical procedure that consists of implanting a device that sends electrical impulses, has been shown helpful in the treatment of Parkinson's disease, chronic pain, depression and obsessive-compulsive disorder.

Despite this new era of technology, neuroscience and psychopharmacology, clinical psychiatrists have gradually changed the more traditional paradigms of care towards a better-balanced biopsychosocial model of care. Today, the importance of psychotherapy, healthy diet and exercise, which can reduce the need for inpatient hospitalization and psychotropic use, has become essential in proper psychiatric care.

As reflected in the film discussions throughout this book, psychiatric themes, psychiatrists and mental illness are very recurrent in the horror genre, and asylums and psychiatry's obsolete treatments provide a perfect setting for a horror film. Soon after the deinstitutionalization movement, in 1972, came British film *Asylum* by Roy Ward Baker. The movie tells the story of Dr. Martin who arrives at the asylum for incurably insane patients to interview for a position as chief doctor. Dr. Martin is received by Dr. Rutherford who as part of the job interview proposes that he talk to four inmates to determine which Dr. Starr is (the former head of the asylum who became insane and is now a patient). Dr. Martin interviews the four patients and learns about their delusions. He concludes that Dr. Starr is a patient who calls himself Dr. Byron and has the ability to transfer his soul to a small automaton with similar facial features. In fact Dr. Byron's automaton is able to escape the room and it kills Dr. Rutherford downstairs. However, Dr. Starr's true identity is Max Reynolds, the assistant at the hospital who, after killing Dr. Martin, continues to interview new candidates for the job. *Asylum* provides four different stories of patients interviewed by Dr. Martin. Voodoo is a central topic. Bonnie, the first patient interviewed by Dr. Martin, recounts how she plotted against Ruth, the wealthy wife of her lover who had knowledge about voodoo. After being killed and cut into pieces, the mutilated parts of her body persecute Bonnie. Dr. Byron has a special power to transfer his soul into an automaton; this practice is also present in voodoo culture. All the patients interviewed by Dr. Martin have psychotic disorders with delusions and hallucinations – positive psychotic symptoms. In contrast, all of them have organized thinking and speech and lack negative psychotic symptoms (lack of spontaneous speech, movement, hygiene, etc.). Symptoms of delusions and hallucinations with outbursts of unpredictable agitation become the stereotype of the dangerous mad patient in asylum horror.

In 1973, S.F. Brownrigg directed the low-budget film *Don't Look in the Basement*. The film is set in a rural sanitarium in which patients are encouraged to act freely on their impulses as part of their innovative therapy. Some of the inmates are a nymphomaniac, a soldier with shell shock (now called PTSD), a lobotomized man, and other patients with severe delusions and disturbance of emotions. With this new approach the situation becomes chaotic and the staff members begin to fear for their own lives.

In the second sequel to *A Nightmare on Elm Street, Dream Warriors* (1987) directed by Chuck Russell, young Kristen's wrists are sliced by Freddy Krueger in a dream but her mother interprets this as a suicide attempt and sends her to a psychiatric ward. There she meets a number of adolescents who suffer the same nightmares about a burnt man. It turns out that all of them are the last children of Elm Street. Nancy – from the first film – is now a staff member who assists Dr. Gordon with these adolescents. Nancy proposes the use of hypnocil, a new experimental drug that helps them stay awake. They also do group hypnotherapy sessions. According to traditional psychoanalysis, dreams are manifestations of the unconscious and therefore the subject of psychoanalytic interpretation. It is believed that through hypnosis a person can access the unconscious and potentially solve a conflicted past. Nancy and Dr. Gordon induce a trance state in these children with the aim of accessing their shared trauma and healing it. Hypnocil, the drug proposed by the Nancy and Dr. Gordon, is a fictional drug. However in real clinical practice, psychiatrists often prescribe modafinil (Provigil) to promote wakefulness in patients with narcolepsy or excessive daytime sleepiness.

With the closing and abandonment of the buildings that hosted the psychiatric asylums, paranormal investigators claimed evidence of the residual activity of the ghosts of the patients who died through the centuries in these institutions. These ideas have inspired a number of TV shows and films. One of them, *Session 9* (2001), is an independent horror film directed by Brad Anderson in which an asbestos removal company, owned by Gordon Fleming, is hired to clean the abandoned Danvers Sanitarium. There the workers find several old icepicks used for lobotomies and nine tapes with the recorded sessions of a patient with dissociative identity disorder, Mary Hobbes. She has two good personalities and an evil one called Simon who pops up in the last session at the same time that we discover Gordon's secret. *Grave Encounters* (2011) by the Vicious Brothers (Colin Minihan and Stuart Ortiz) is a found footage-style film in which a group of skeptical paranormal investigators suffer attacks from the ghosts and spirits of the patients that inhabited Collingwood Psychiatric Hospital. The second season of the popular TV show *American Horror Story: Asylum* (2012–13) presents a number of horror film clichés and stereotypes about mental illness.

In the field of psychiatry, there is a debate about whether horror films and in particular those that bring specific psychiatric themes onto the screen stigmatize psychiatry and mental illness. A recent article published in *The Lancet Psychiatry* proposes several ideas to avoid stigma, such as the use of disclaimers stating that the depictions of mental illness are fictional. Nonetheless, the general basis of cinema is to portray unrealistic settings that allow the spectator to escape reality. In horror cinema, insanity and fear of becoming mad or being locked up in an asylum are common themes. The distortion of reality maximizes the fearful feeling. For the most part, as in the other film genres, in horror films the audience will know the difference between movies and real life.

CHAPTER 14

Psychiatry and Horror

"CATHARSIS" WAS A TERM defined by Aristotle (384–322 BCE) in his *Poetics* to refer to the purging or purification of emotions when watching tragedy or pity. The catharsis theory of art and cinema supports the relief or pleasure of the audience when watching a film that elicits certain emotions. Congruent with the catharsis theory, films have traditionally been classified under several genres depending on the intended emotion elicited in the viewer. Therefore a romantic film will draw out feelings of love, an action film provokes tension, comedy can induce laughter, tragedy can produce sorrow and the success of horror will depend on the potential to cause fear in the audience. Congruent with this catharsis theory, Stephen King asserts that horror acts as a sort of safety valve for our cruel or aggressive impulses. Psychoanalyst Glen O. Gabbard states that horror films allow the spectator to evoke inner fears but with a sense of control. For Sigmund Freud, monsters, freaks and demons represent the unknown, what is not familiar to us. They are representations of our id, our repressed impulses that are perceived as threatening by our superego which, due to a symbolic fear of castration, attempts to repress what is not accepted by society. In that sense, monsters and demons are blamed for calamities.

From an evolutional perspective, since the beginning of our existence humans have faced fears of being devoured by a beast in the middle of the night, being bitten by spiders or snakes, or falling off a cliff. According to the imprinting theory of Konrad Lorenz, some of the behaviors to defend against this threat were congenitally imprinted at birth. A clear example of this kind of congenital fright is the fear of loud noises. Every child has it and it may have served as an adaptive survival skill. In addition, research shows that little children show a tendency to experience more fear when faced with the image of a threatening animal than with a bloody knife. This concept was also referred to by Carl Jung as our collective unconscious. Many of us may have never seen a snake or spider but are still susceptible of developing a phobia to these creatures. In addition, the feared objects vary historically depending on the social context. For example, as explained in earlier chapters, a fear of an invasion was common during the Cold War, which explains the success of films about alien invaders from outer space. Nowadays, with the memory of the recent financial crisis, a fear of system collapse would explain the success of zombie and apocalyptic films.

The feeling of fear is often accompanied by excitement, which would further explain the joy that we experience when watching a horror film. Physiologically, when people experience fear generally and when they are watching horrific images, they experience an increase in the heart rate and blood pressure, muscle tension, sweating, and a lowering of the skin temperature. Our adrenal glands secrete adrenaline, a hormone and neurotransmitter that enhances our feeling of excitement. In addition, endorphins, endogenous neuropeptides that invoke euphoria, are released by our brain in situations of stress, pain and fear. These mechanisms support a sensation-seeking theory of why people like horror.

Fear is an innate emotion needed for survival. Anatomically, most research studies show the amygdala, a group of neurons in the deep brain medial to the temporal lobe, as the most relevant structure in our brain for the mediation of fear. Studies performed on war veterans with damage in their amygdalae show a lack of fear response and no incidence of PTSD. According to neuroscience fear is first perceived by our senses (such as visual, auditory, tactile) and travels to the thalamus (a common pathway to all sensory pathways) which signals to the amygdala to activate the fear response, classically a fight, flight or freeze response. The thalamus also sends sensory inputs to the cortex (our conscious brain), particularly to the prefrontal cortex (in charge of the executive functions, in other words the ability to make a decision and a plan). The prefrontal cortex will therefore determine how threatening the feared object is, increasing or decreasing the fear response and making a plan of action. For example, if a person is swimming at the beach and sees a white mass floating, the visual pathways will send inputs to the thalamus about a possible danger (such as a jellyfish) and activate a flight response. In a very short time, the cortex may interpret the white mass as something not threatening (like a plastic bag) and the person may decide to continue swimming pleasantly. To make this kind of decision, the prefrontal cortex will also receive inputs from the areas of the brain related to our own memory that allow the integration of all the information (the parietal-temporal-occipital cortex and the hippocampus). The formation of memories in our brain is mediated by the excitatory neurotransmitter glutamate that activates NMDA receptors. In fact, D-cycloserine (previously used as an antibiotic against tuberculosis) activates NMDA receptors, enhancing the ability for learning in cognitive therapy and helping fear extinction in patients with PTSD and social anxiety.

These circuits give us a general idea of how fear is mediated in our brain. As neuroscience continues to progress, we will better understand the role of the neurotransmitters and other areas of the brain in the mechanism of fear. These pathways can also vary depending on the context and situation. In 2010, in a study published in *Human Brain Mapping* by Thomas Straube and colleagues, the brains of forty subjects who were exposed to neutral and scary scenes from horror movies were imaged. They found that threat scenes induced increased activation in the anterior cingulate cortex, insular cortex, thalamus, and visual areas. Whereas the thalamus and the visual cortex are needed for processing the information of watching a film, the insular cortex helps the display of conscious emotions and the anterior cingulate cortex mediates empathy (which allows the viewer to empathize with the situation that the protagonist may be facing). The anterior cingulate cortex also mediates impulse control and regulates the autonomic system (as a result our heart rate, blood pressure, breathing, bowel and other vagal functions can be activated by our experience of watching a horror movie). Furthermore, according to Straube's findings, patients who had movie-induced anxiety had more activation in the dorsomedial prefrontal cortex, an important area of the brain for social processing and understanding another person's preferences. For the authors, the dorsomedial prefrontal cortex had a role in the subjective experience of being scared.

The anatomical areas mentioned allow humans to have theory of mind; that's to say the intuitive understanding of one's own and other people's minds and mental states (thoughts, beliefs, perceptions, emotions, motivations, and so on). Theory of mind is needed to understand the experience of a different person and empathize with it. Thus, theory of mind is needed to understand and feel an emotion when watching a horror film. Theory of mind allows humans to see themselves, whether in the past when they were children or in the future when they become old, as unique entities and understand that at some point in their existence, like every other human being, they will face their ultimate fear, death. Horror reflects an existentialist approach to life and death. Existentialism is a philosophical movement that emphasizes human responsibility and freedom of choice in determining their own development through the acts of their will. In existentialism as in most horror films, there is no life after death; the victims don't go to heaven. Therefore, at the same time that horror offers a catharsis to death anxiety, it stimulates the importance of focusing on life in the present and encourages us to enjoy life and to experience the pleasures that it offers. As a result, it is not surprising that comedy and eroticism are recurrent themes in horror films. In a philosophical way, horror films can awaken our angst towards the authentic experience of our own existence.

References and Further Reading

American Psychiatric Association (APA) (2013). *Diagnostic and Statistical Manual of Mental Disorders: DSM-5*. 5th ed. Arlington, VA: APA.

Aristotle (1987). *Poetics*. Indianapolis, IN: Hackett Pub. Co.

Bongar, Bruce and Beutler, Larry E. (1995). *Comprehensive Textbook of Psychotherapy: Theory and Practice*. Oxford: Oxford University Press.

Breitbart, William and Poppitto, Shannon (2014). *Individual Meaning-Centered Psychotherapy in Patients with Advanced Cancer*. Oxford: Oxford University Press.

Brooks, Max (2003). *The Zombie Survival Guide: Complete Protection from the Living Dead*. New York: Broadway Books.

Brown, Mathew (2013). *The Evil Dead* by Sam Raimi, *The Journal of Humanistic Psychiatry*. 1(4): 24–25.

Caesar, J. (1982). *The Conquer of The Gaul*. London: Penguin Books.

Camus, Albert (1991). *The Myth of Sisyphus and Other Essays*. New York: Vintage.

Carrol, Noel (1990). *The Philosophy of Horror or Paradoxes of the Heart*. New York: Routledge.

Centers for Disease Control and Prevention (CDC) (2016). *Rabies*. Available online at: www.cdc.gov/rabies/

Centers for Disease Control and Prevention (CDC) (2011). *Recovery of a Patient from Clinical Rabies — California*, 2011. Available online at: www.cdc.gov/mmwr/preview/ mmwrhtml/mm6104a1.htm

Dein, Simon and Littlewood, Robert (2011). Religion and psychosis: a common evolutionary trajectory?, *Transcultural Psychiatry*. 48(3): 318–35.

Eisner, Lotte H. (1969). *The Haunted Screen; expressionism in the German cinema and the influence of Max Reinhardt*. Berkeley, CA: University of California.

Espi Forcen, Carlos (2015). Future humans: speculations towards the future of humans in Michel Houellebecq, *The Journal of Humanistic Psychiatry*. 3(4): 10–14.

Espi Forcen, Carlos (2013). The triumph of death in Late Medieval Italian painting, *The Journal of Humanistic Psychiatry*. 1(2): 10–12.

Espi Forcen, Carlos (2013). Trance and mental pathologies in 20th century art, *The Journal of Humanistic Psychiatry*. 1(4): 8–12.

Espi Forcen, Carlos (2014). Fake accusations for real aggressions: the blood libel against the Jews in the Late Middle Ages, *The Journal of Humanistic Psychiatry*. 2(4): 10–14.

Espi Forcen, Carlos (2014). Medieval anxiety and the anxiety towards the alien, *The Journal of Humanistic Psychiatry*. 2(1): 13–18.

Espi Forcen, Carlos and Espi Forcen, Fernando (2014). Demonic possessions and mental illness: discussion of selected cases in Late Medieval hagiographical literature, *Early Science and Medicine*. 10(3): 258–79.

Espi Forcen, Fernando (2013). Between life and death: the phenomenology of near death experiences, *The Journal of Humanistic Psychiatry*. 1(2): 13–14.

Espi Forcen, Fernando (2013). *Doctor Caligari* and *The Somnambulist*, *The Journal of Humanistic Psychiatry*. 1(4): 5.

Espi Forcen, Fernando (2013). Psychiatry and American horror film sagas, *The Journal of Humanistic Psychiatry*. 1(4): 6–7.

Espi Forcen, Fernando (2013). Sex, rock and psychedelia, *The Journal of Humanistic Psychiatry*. 1(3): 15–17.

Espi Forcen, Fernando (2013). *The Exorcist* by William Friedkin, *The Journal of Humanistic Psychiatry*. 1(4): 23–24.

Espi Forcen, Fernando (2013). The voodoo practice and the zombie problem of human existence, *The Journal of Humanistic Psychiatry*. 1(4): 18–21.

Espi Forcen, Fernando (2013). Trance states, *The Journal of Humanistic Psychiatry*. 1(4): 4.

Espi Forcen, Fernando (2014). Aggression and narcissism, *The Journal of Humanistic Psychiatry*. 2(4): 4–6.

Espi Forcen, Fernando (2014). Aliens from outer space: the human obsession with the search for life on other planets and its existential consequences. *The Journal of Humanistic Psychiatry*. 2(1): 19–22.

Espi Forcen, Fernando (2014). Aquelarre (Witches' Sabbath), *The Journal of Humanistic Psychiatry*. 2(1): 5–6.

Espi Forcen, Fernando (2014). Cronenberg's *The Fly* and its parallels with Kafka's *Metamorphosis*, *The Journal of Humanistic Psychiatry*. 2(2): 28–29.

Espi Forcen, Fernando (2014). Towards humanism in psychosis, *The Journal of Humanistic Psychiatry*. 2(1): 4.

Espi Forcen, Fernando (2015). Oral pleasure, *The Journal of Humanistic Psychiatry*. 3(2): 4–5.

Espi Forcen, Fernando (2015). Psychiatry and free will, *The Journal of Humanistic Psychiatry*. (3)1: 12–14.

Espi Forcen, Fernando (2015). The meaning of dreams, *The Journal of Humanistic Psychiatry*. 3(4): 19–21.

Espi Forcen, Fernando (2015). The origin of human consciousness, *The Journal of Humanistic Psychiatry*. 3(4): 6–7.

Espi Forcen, Fernando (2015). William Stoughton's shame avoidance at the Salem Witch Trials, *The Journal of Humanistic Psychiatry*. 3(3): 15–20.

Espi Forcen, Fernando and Espi Forcen, Carlos (2015). The practice of holy fasting in the Late Middle Ages: a psychiatric approach, *Journal of Nervous and Mental Diseases*. 203(8): 650–53.

Espi Forcen, Fernando and Espi Forcen, Carlos (2016). *Ars Moriendi*: coping with death in the Late Middle Ages, *Palliative and Supportive Care*. December 15, 2015.

Espi Forcen, Fernando, Hatters Friedman, Susan and Shand, John P. (2014). *American Horror Film and Psychiatry*, workshop at the 167th APA Annual Meeting, May 3–7, New York, NY.

Espi Rubio, Sergio (2014). The trap of romantic love in cinema, *The Journal of Humanistic Psychiatry*. 2(2): 15–18.

Foucault, Michel (1965). *Madness and Civilization*. New York: Random House.

Freud, Sigmund (1905; 2000). *Three Essays on the Theory of Sexuality*. New York: Basic Books.

Freud, Sigmund (1913; 1989). *Totem and Taboo*. New York: Routledge and Kegan Paul.

Freud, Sigmund (1914; 2010). *The Wolfman*. New York: Penguin Great Ideas.

Freud, Sigmund (1919; 2003). *The Uncanny*. New York: Penguin Books.

Freud, Sigmund (1958; 1990). *On Dreams*. New York: Norton & Company.

Gabbard, Glenn O. and Gabbard, Krin (1999). *Psychiatry and the Cinema*. Arlington, VA: American Psychiatric Publishing.

Hales, Robert E., Yudofsky, Stuart C. and Robert, Laura Weiss (2014). *The American Psychiatric Publishing Textbook of Psychiatry*. Arlington, VA: American Psychiatric Publishing.

Harris, Sam (2012). *Free Will*. New York: Free Press.

Hatters Friedman, Susan, Espi Forcen, Fernando and Shand, John Preston (2014). Horror films and psychiatry, *Australasian Psychiatry*. 22(5): 447–49.

Hatters Friedman, Susan, McCue Horwitz, S. and Resnick, P. (2005). Child murder by mothers: a clear analysis of the current state of knowledge and a research agenda, *American Journal of Psychiatry*. 162(9): 1578–87.

Heidegger, Martin (1927; 2008). *Being and Time*. New York: Harper Perennial Modern Classics.

Hendershot, Cynthia (1999). *Paranoia, the Bomb and the 1950s Scientific Films*. Bowling Green, OH: Bowling Green University Press.

Holland, J. (ed.) (2015). *Psycho-oncology*. Oxford: Oxford University Press.

Houellebecq, M. (2005). *The Possibility of an Island*. New York: Alfred A. Knopf.

Hubner, Laura, Leaning, Marcus and Manning, Paul (2015). *The Zombie Renaissance in Popular Culture*. New York: Palgrave Macmillan.

Indick, William (2004). *Movies and The Mind: Theory of The Great Psychoanalysts Applied to Film*. Jefferson, NC: McFarland.

Irwing, Harvery J. and Watt, Caroline A. (2007). *An Introduction to Parapsychology*. Jefferson, NC: McFarland.

Isenberg, Noah (2009). *Weimar Cinema: An Essential Guider to Classic Films of the Era*. New York: Columbia University Press.

Jung, Carl G. (1981). *The Archetypes and The Collective Unconscious*. Princeton, NJ: Princeton University Press.

Kant, I. (2007). *Critique of Pure Reason*. London: Penguin.

Kaufman, Myland (2013). *Kaufman's Clinical Neurology for Psychiatrists*. St Louis, MO: Saunders.

Klein, M. (1988). *Love, Guilt and Reparation*. London: Virago.

Kramer, Heinrich (1486; 1971). *Malleus Maleficarum*. Mineola, NY: Dover Occult.

Lacan, Jacques (2009). *My Teaching*. New York: Verso.

Lilly, John C. (1972). *The Center of The Cyclone: An Autobiography of Inner Space*. New York: Julian Press.

Marcus Aurelius (2015). *Meditations*. London: Penguin Classics.

Packer, Sharon (2012). *Cinema's Sinister Psychiatrists: From Caligari to Hannibal*. Jefferson, NC: McFarland.

Perkins, Franklin (2016). *The Greatest Mistake: Teleology, Anthropomorphism and the Rise of Science*. Under review (source: Academia.edu).

Phillips, Kendall R. (2005). *Projected Fears: Horror Films and American Culture*. Westport, CT: Praeger.

Plato (2000). *The Republic*. Cambridge: Cambridge University Press.

Pope, Stephanie. (2013). Philippe Pinel (1745–1826): more that the liberator of the insane, *Journal of Humanistic Psychiatry*. 1(1): 12–13.

Purves, Dale, Augustine, George J., Fitzpatrick, David, Hall, William C., Lamantia, Anthony-Samuel and White, Leonard E. (2011). *Neuroscience*. Sunderland, MA: Sinauer Associates.

Riches, Simon (2012). *The Philosophy of David Cronenberg (Philosophy of Popular Culture)*. Lexington, KY: University Press of Kentucky.

Robinson, David (2003). *Reel Psychiatry: Movie Portrayals of Psychiatric Conditions*. Port Huron, MI: Rapid Psychler.

Russell, Jeffrey B. and Alexander, Brooks (2007). *A History of Witchcraft: Sorcerers, Heretics and Pagans*. London: Thames & Hudson.

Rutter, Michael (ed.) (2010). *Rutter's Child and Adolescent Psychiatry 5th Edition*. Oxford: Wiley-Blackwell.

Sadock, Benjamin James, Sadock, Virginia Alcott and Ruiz, Pedro (2009). *Kaplan and Sadock's Comprehensive Textbook of Psychiatry*. Philadelphia, PA: Lippincott Williams and Wilkins.

Saint Thomas Aquinas (1981). *Summa Theologica*. Westminster, MD: Thomas More Publishing.

Sartre, Jean-Paul (1943; 1993). *Being and Nothingness*. New York: Washington Square Press.

Sartre, Jean-Paul (1945; 2007). *Existentialism is a Humanism*. New Haven, CT: Yale University Press.

Schlozman, Steven C. (2012). *The Zombie Autopsies: Secret Notebooks from the Apocalypse*. New York: Grand Central Publishing.

Schopenhauer, Arthur (1966). *The World as Will and Representation*. Mineola, NY: Dover Publications.

Sears, Kathleen (2014). *Greek Mythology 101: From Gods and Goddesses to Monsters and Mortals*. Avon, MA: Adams Media.

Seneca (2005). *On The Shortness of Life*. New York: Penguin Books.

Shand, John Preston, Hatters Friedman, Susan and Espi Forcen, Fernando (2014). The horror, the horror: stigma on screen, *Lancet Psychiatry*. 31(1): 423–24.

Sherman, Aubrey (2014). *Vampires: The Myths, Legends and Lore*. Avon, MA: Adams Media.

Shorter, Edward (1998). *A History of Psychiatry: From the Era of the Asylum to the Age of Prozac*. Hoboken, NJ: Wiley.

Sophocles (1978). *Oedipus The King*. New York: Oxford University.

Sophocles (1953). *Electra*. London: Penguin Books.

Stanford Encyclopedia of Philosophy. Available online at: http://plato.stanford.edu/

Straube, Thomas, Preissler, Sandra, Lipka, Judith, Hewig, Johannes, Mentzel, Hans-Joachim and Miltner, Wolfgang H.R. (2010). Neural representation of anxiety and personality during exposure to anxiety-provoking and neutral scenes from scary movies, *Human Brain Mapping*. 31(1): 36–47.

Thaker, Eugene (2011). *In the Dust of This Planet: Horror of Philosophy vol. 1*. Alresford: Zero Books.

Trigg, Dylan (2014). *The Thing: A Phenomenology of Horror*. Alresford: Zero Books.

Tudor, Andrew (1989). *Monsters and Mad Scientists: A Cultural History of the Horror Movies*. Oxford: Basil Blackwell.

Wasik, Bill and Murphy, Monica (2013). *Rabid: A Cultural History of the World's Most Diabolical Virus*. New York: Penguin.

Wedding, Danny, Niemiec, Ryan M. (2014). *Movies and Mental Illness*. Boston, MA: Hogrefe Publishing.

Wein, Simon (2015). Between space and consciousness – the final frontier, *The Journal of Humanistic Psychiatry*. 3(4): 22–32.

Worland, Rick (2007). *The Horror Film: An Introduction*. Malden, MA: Blackwell.

Žižek, Slavoj (2006). *The Pervert's Guide to Cinema*. Documentary. Director: Sophie Fiennes. Mischief Films/Amoeba Films.

Index